Anatomy of the Forehead, Face, and Neck

Edward H. Bedrossian Jr., MD, FACS
Richard R. Schmidt, PhD
Robert C. Della Rocca, MD, FACS
Bradley N. Lemke, MD, FACS
Editors

Anatomy of the Forehead, Face, and Neck

A Dissection Manual

Springer

Editors
Edward H. Bedrossian Jr., MD, FACS
Wills Eye Hospital
Philadelphia, PA, USA

Robert C. Della Rocca, MD, FACS (Deceased)
Icahn School of Medicine
New York Eye and Ear Infirmary
New York, NY, USA

Richard R. Schmidt, PhD (Deceased)
Sydney Kimmel Medical College
Thomas Jefferson University
Philadelphia, PA, USA

Bradley N. Lemke, MD, FACS
School of Medicine and Public Health
University of Wisconsin System
Madison, WI, USA

ISBN 978-3-031-56142-9   ISBN 978-3-031-56140-5 (eBook)
https://doi.org/10.1007/978-3-031-56140-5

This Springer imprint is published by the registered company Springer Nature Switzerland AG
The registered company address is: Gewerbestrasse 11, 6330 Cham, Switzerland
Paper in this product is recyclable.

To my Grandfather, Edward H. Bedrossian, MD, for his philanthropy and compassion since 1924, as one of the very first ophthalmologists.
To my Father, E. Howard Bedrossian, MD, for his guidance, passion, and pursuit of quality care.
To my wife, Iryna, for her ever-present love and support.
To Wills Eye Hospital and Temple Ophthalmology Department, for their commitment to excellence in clinical care, resident education, and research.

Edward H. Bedrossian, Jr., MD, FACS

I owe an unimaginable amount of gratitude to my best friend and wife, Dulcie, for her never-ending support and encouragement for this work and throughout my career. All of my children, Allison, Garret, Robert, and Ryan, and their spouses, Jon, Katie, Ashley, and Lisa, are more than deserving of considerable praise and thanks for their patience, understanding, and continued support over the years. The final portion of this dedication is to our seven grandchildren, Jack, Sofia, Lizzie, Ella, Bryson, Joie, and Matthew, as well as to my present and former students who have made this educational experience remarkably fulfilling.

Richard R. Schmidt, PhD

I wish to express gratitude to my ever-supportive wife Gale and loving family, and I thank Richard K. Dortzbach, MD, and Orkan George Stasior, MD, for sharing with me their passion for the anatomy.

Bradley N. Lemke, MD, FACS

Foreword

There is a reason why medical school commences with the exploration of a cadaver in the anatomy lab: a profound understanding of the human body's anatomy forms the foundation of medical practice. Nowhere is this truer than in the realm of facial plastic surgery, where an in-depth comprehension of facial anatomy is indispensable. With great enthusiasm, the authors present *Anatomy of the Forehead, Face, and Neck: A Dissection Manual*, a work that promises immense value to a myriad of surgical specialists, including ophthalmologists, plastic surgeons, otolaryngologists, dermatologists, and maxillofacial surgeons. Medical students embarking on the journey of facial anatomy exploration will find this manual to be an invaluable companion.

Within these pages lies a treasure trove of information about anatomical structures that have long piqued the curiosity of medical practitioners and students alike. Ever wondered about Yasargil's fat pad and its relationship to the frontal branch of the facial nerve? Or the anatomy of the platysma muscle and the triangles of the neck? Moreover, you will find insights into the significance of the orbitomalar ligament and the temporal line of fusion. This manual meticulously addresses these topics and more, illustrated by informative dissections and helpful illustrations, bringing clarity to the many aspects of facial anatomy. The clinical correlations are especially useful.

The collaborative effort of the four authors is a testament to their passion for anatomy. Each possesses an abiding fascination with the subject, evident in their combined decades of experience teaching anatomical dissection courses. Their dedication has left an indelible mark on the educational paths of many medical students and healthcare professionals, nurturing an enduring appreciation for the significance of anatomy in medical practice.

As you delve into the intricacies of facial anatomy through this manual, may you be inspired by the wisdom and expertise of these accomplished authors. I am confident that *Anatomy of the Forehead, Face, and Neck: A Dissection Manual* will serve as an indispensable guide and will foster a deeper understanding of the anatomy that underlies the art and science of facial plastic surgery.

University of Colorado Health Sciences Center
Denver, Colorado, USA

Michael John Hawes

In Memory of Dr. Richard R. Schmidt

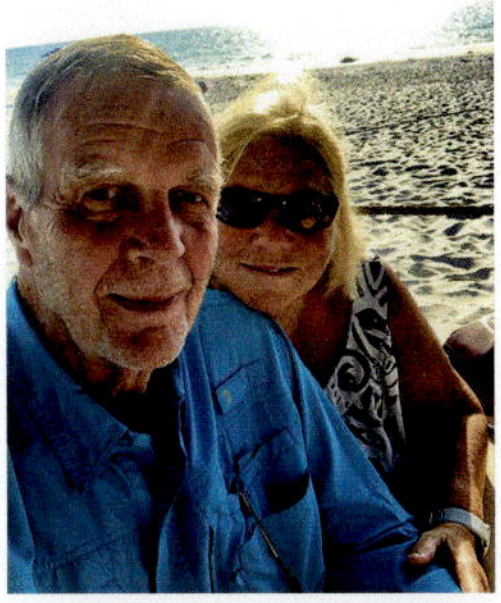

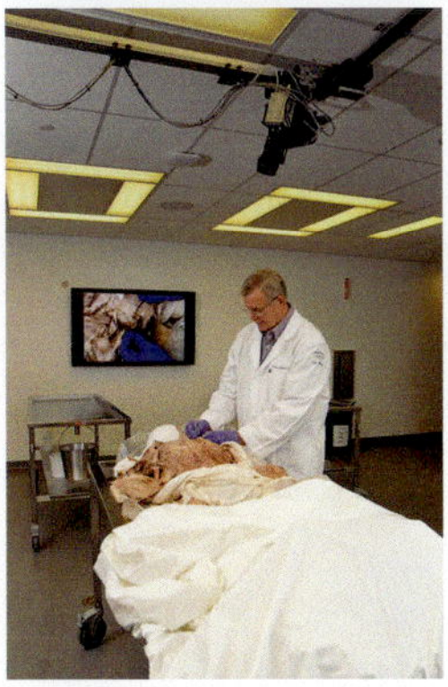

This collaborative tribute honors the remarkable Dr. Richard R. Schmidt, whose passion for knowledge shaped a distinguished 48-year tenure at Sidney Kimmel Medical College. Unfortunately, he passed away shortly before the text was published and did not see the final version. The tribute is co-written by his beloved wife Dulcie and son, Ryan.

Dr. Schmidt made enduring contributions to embryology, gross anatomy, histology, and neuroscience education.

Recipient of esteemed teaching awards, including the Lindback Foundation award, Dr. Schmidt's influence went beyond the classroom, impacting more than 10,000 medical professionals. His legacy, celebrated here, reflects unwavering commitment to excellence and a passion for lifelong learning.

Farewell to a remarkable educator, mentor, and family man. Dr. Richard R. Schmidt is remembered for love, kindness, and wisdom. His enduring legacy, alongside dedicated educators like Drs. Bedrossian, Della Rocca, and Lemke, continues to shape medical education.

Survived by his loving wife, Dulcie Schmidt, and children, Allison, Garrett, Robert, and Ryan, Richard's legacy lives on through cherished grandchildren. In addition to teaching, he found solace in fishing, aviary photography, and snowboarding, creating lasting memories with his beloved family.

Preface

There are many outstanding textbooks on the anatomy of the Forehead, Face, and Neck. This manual is an aide for the Ophthalmologist and Oculofacial Plastic surgeon learning the complexities of this anatomy and is not a substitute for a fellowship in Oculo-Facial Plastic Surgery. The Plastic Surgeon, ENT Facial Plastic Surgeon, Cosmetic Surgeon, or Dermatologic Surgeon will also benefit from this dissection manual, but there are more detailed dissection manuals for each specialty.

This manual is similar to its companion *Anatomy of the Eyelid, Orbit, and Lacrimal System: A Dissection Manual* (Springer, 2022) in that it presents a step-by-step dissection in a layered approach, clarifying the complex anatomy of the soft tissues.

This method of facial anatomic study began in 1983 at the New York Eye and Ear Infirmary. Robert Della Rocca, MD, invited Bradley Lemke, MD, to create and present an orbital anatomy dissection method in New York. It was taught with Edward H. Bedrossian Jr., MD, then the Ophthalmic Plastic Surgery Fellow. The periorbital area is covered in the first of this two-volume set. With the expansion of Ophthalmic Plastic and Reconstructive Surgery into the Forehead, Face, and Neck, this second volume reflects the continuing facial anatomy dissection and surgical experience of the authors.

Special emphasis has been given to forehead and facelifting surgical anatomy. This manual differs from the first in that each chapter has an optional "surgical dissection" section. Once appreciative of the three-dimensional anatomic layers, the student will benefit from the cosmetic "surgical dissection," which crosses anatomic planes. The "surgical dissection" requires a second cadaver and represents one of many surgical approaches.

This manual, which is enhanced with more illustrations and expert contributors, consists of four chapters. Chapter 1 describes how the specimens are prepared and stored. Chapter 2 describes dissection of the Forehead and Eyebrows. Chapter 3, the largest chapter, describes dissection of the Midface, Nose, Ear, and Lower Face. Chapter 4 describes dissection of the Neck. To maximize the use of each specimen, it is recommended to follow the chapters sequentially.

In 1984, Dr. Bedrossian, Director of the Wills Eye Hospital Annual Resident Orbital Dissection Course, met Richard R. Schmidt, PhD, then Associate Professor of Anatomy, Pathology, and Cell Biology. Over the next 40 years, without interruption even during the 2020 Covid pandemic, they developed and refined an instructional course that is regarded at Wills Eye Hospital as one of the most important of their residency.

The course has been presented with updates and expansions in scope over 120 times at Wills Eye Hospital, at the University of Wisconsin-Madison, and at the American Academy of Ophthalmology Annual Meetings. It is estimated that more than 2000 ophthalmology residents, oculofacial plastic fellows, and international physicians have benefited from the courses, which follow the step-by-step approach outlined in these manuals. The manuals may be used alone or as complements.

We are pleased to have Michael J. Hawes, MD, a leader in Oculofacial Plastic Surgery and past president of the American Society of Ophthalmic Plastic and Reconstructive Surgery (ASPORS), accept our invitation to write the Foreword. Dr. Hawes is a recognized anatomist, who has published award-winning research. He shares our enthusiasm in this manual written by oculofacial plastic surgeons for ophthalmologists and oculofacial plastic surgeons, head and neck surgeons, plastic surgeons, and cosmetic surgeons interested in cosmetic surgery of the eyelids, forehead, face, and neck.

Philadelphia, PA, USA — Edward H. Bedrossian Jr., MD, FACS
Philadelphia, PA, USA — Richard R. Schmidt, PhD
New York, NY, USA — Robert C. Della Rocca, MD, FACS
Madison, WI, USA — Bradley N. Lemke, MD, FACS

Acknowledgments

A Dissection Manual of this nature is the result of the tireless efforts of so many people. First, we remember Robert C. Della Rocca, MD, FACS, who was so inspirational for the companion manual, *Anatomy of the Eyelid, Orbit, and Lacrimal System: A Dissection Manual*, published by Springer in 2022. Those studying this manual will be the beneficiary of his legendary passion for teaching surgical anatomy.

We thank Bradley N. Lemke, MD, FACS, for his expertise, interest, and increased contribution to this manual. We appreciate the dedication and intense time spent in the anatomy laboratory by our outstanding Wills Eye Hospital Oculofacial Plastic surgeons Sathyadeepak Ramesh, MD, and Alison Watson, MD, FACS, as well as Wills Eye Hospital Oculofacial Plastic fellow Karine Shebaclo, MD.

As with the first manual *Anatomy of the Eyelid, Orbit and Lacrimal System: A Dissection Manual*, this manual would not have been possible without the unyielding support of Dr. Schmidt and the assistance of Philip (Chris) Marcucci, the Dissection Coordinator at Sidney Kimmel Medical College of Thomas Jefferson University for the procurement and preparation of specimens under Dr. Schmidt's supervision.

The editors are indebted to the professional illustrators at Springer for their beautiful artwork and Lee Klein (Senior Editor) for his enthusiasm and persistence in bringing this manual to completion.

Contents

Contributors

Edward H. Bedrossian Jr., MD, FACS Wills Eye Hospital, Sydney Kimmel Medical College of Thomas Jefferson University, Philadelphia, PA, USA

Department of Oculoplastic and Orbital Surgery, Wills Eye Hospital, Philadelphia, PA, USA

Clinical Professor Ophthalmology, Lewis Katz School of Medicine at Temple University, Philadelphia, PA, USA

Oculo-Facial Plastics Department, Wills Eye Hospital, Philadelphia, PA, USA

Clinical Professor Ophthalmology, Oculofacial Plastic Orbital Reconstructive Surgery, Lewis Katz School of Medicine at Temple University, Philadelphia, PA, USA

Robert C. Della Rocca, MD, FACS Icahn School of Medicine, New York Eye and Ear Infirmary, New York, NY, USA

Michael John Hawes, MD, FACS Department of Ophthalmology, University of Colorado Health Sciences Center, Denver, CO, USA

Bradley N. Lemke, MD, FACS Lemke Facial Surgery, Madison, WI, USA

Department of Ophthalmology and Visual Sciences, School of Medicine and Public Health, University of Wisconsin-Madison, Madison, WI, USA

Sathyadeepak Ramesh, MD The Center for Eye and Facial Plastic Surgery, Somerset, NJ, USA

Richard R. Schmidt, PhD Department of Pathology, Anatomy and Cell Biology, Sydney Kimmel Medical College of Thomas Jefferson University, Philadelphia, PA, USA

Kareen Shebaclo, MD Department of Oculoplastic and Orbital Surgery, Wills Eye Hospital, Philadelphia, PA, USA

Alison H. Watson, MD, FACS Department of Oculoplastic and Orbital Surgery, Wills Eye Hospital, Philadelphia, PA, USA

Cadaver Preparation and Embalming Procedure

1

Richard R. Schmidt

Introduction

The preparation of specimens is a vital component of any dissection course. Thus, this first chapter describes how the cadavers are disinfected, prepared, embalmed, and subsequently stored prior to and during utilization.

Refrigeration is always recommended after death. Cadaver should be embalmed within 48 h following death for optimal results.

Once clothing is removed as well as feeding tubes, IV lines, etc., the entire body is disinfected with Dis-Spray purchased from Hydrol Chemical. Mouth and nasal cavity are sprayed with Dis-Spray or Oral-Balm also from Hydrol Chemical. Next the entire body is washed with soap and hot water.

An incision is then made superior to the clavicle along the medial border of the sternocleidomastoid muscle. This approach follows the groove between the trachea and the carotid sheath. Remove the fascia of the carotid sheath and expose the internal jugular vein and the carotid artery. Make a small cut in the artery, but do not cut all the way through. Use two pieces of string each about 8 in. long around the artery about 1 in. apart. Insert one injection canula down toward the heart and the other upward toward the head. Tighten the strings around each canula. Make a small cut in the internal jugular vein and insert a drain tube.

We typically use a pre-injection fluid (Fig. 1.1), Saturol (Hydrol Chemical). First mix 32 oz of Saturol with 2 gallons of water. Connect embalming machine (Fig. 1.2) hose to canula and with pressure set at 10 PSI inject ½ gallon up toward head and remainder down toward heart.

We are now ready to inject the embalming fluid (Fig. 1.3). The fluid we use is the Maryland Solution (Hydrol Chemical). It has the following components: Glycerin (33.3%), Phenol (27.8%), 37% Formaldehyde (5.6%), and Methanol (33.3%). One-part Maryland Solution is mixed with two parts water. Connect embalming machine hose to canula up toward head, set pressure at 20 PSI and inject about 1 gallon. Remove hose from the up canula and place on the down canula injecting the remainder of the fluid. Mix another three gallons of the embalming fluid and

Richard R. Schmidt has died before the publication of this book.

R. R. Schmidt, PhD (Deceased) (✉)
Department of Pathology, Anatomy and Cell Biology, Sydney Kimmel Medical College of Thomas Jefferson University, Philadelphia, PA, USA

E. H. Bedrossian Jr et al. (eds.), *Anatomy of the Forehead, Face, and Neck*,
https://doi.org/10.1007/978-3-031-56140-5_1

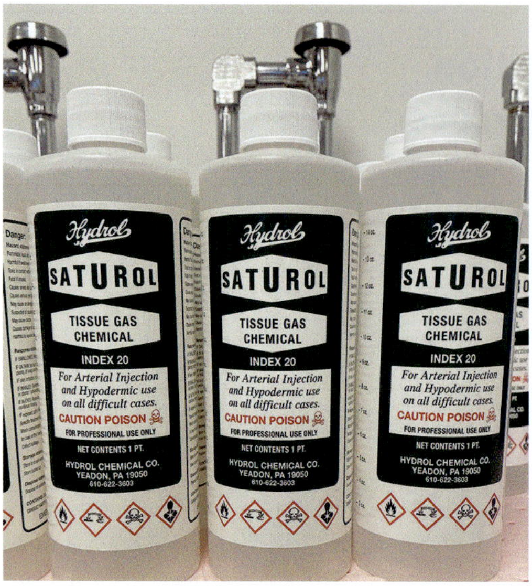

Fig. 1.1 Saturol, pre-injection fluid

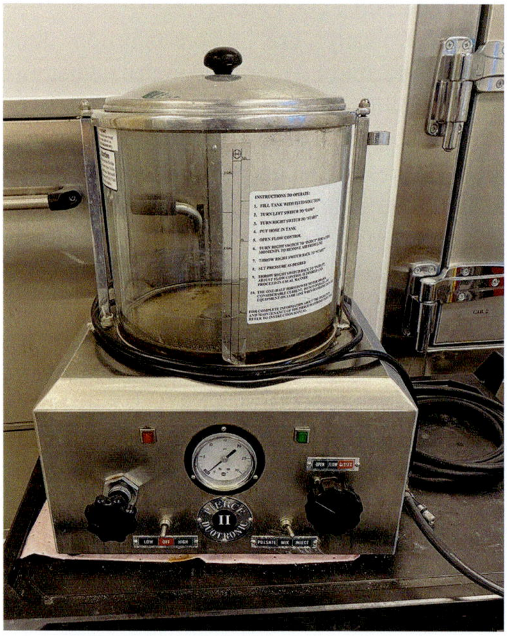

Fig. 1.2 Embalming machine

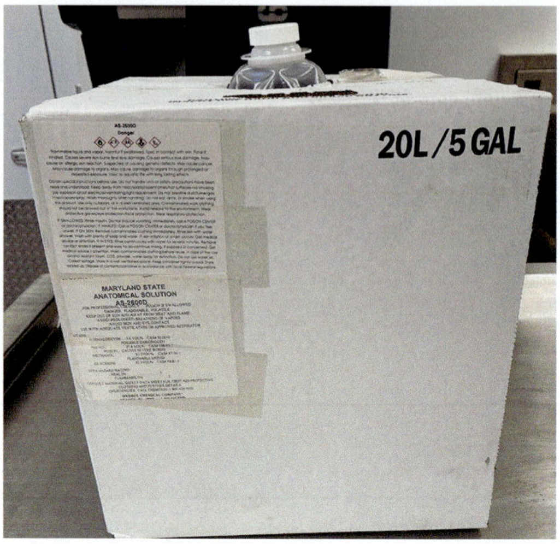

Fig. 1.3 Maryland solution

continue to inject downward toward heart. Keep watch on the drain tube in the internal jugular vein ensuring a continuous flow of blood which will change from bright red to orange as the fluid is distributed throughout the body. You should visually note changes such as swelling of embalmed areas, skin change to white and firming of the body. If there is any doubt about proper distribution of the fluid, arteries in the arms and lower limbs may be raised for injection. The axillary artery and femoral artery are recommended for these injections.

The cadaver is covered with plastic sheeting and allowed to drain for 3 or 4 days a room temperature. Typically, the brain is then removed and placed in formalin. The cadaver is then placed in a plastic bag and transferred to refrigerated (not frozen) storage until use (Fig. 1.4).

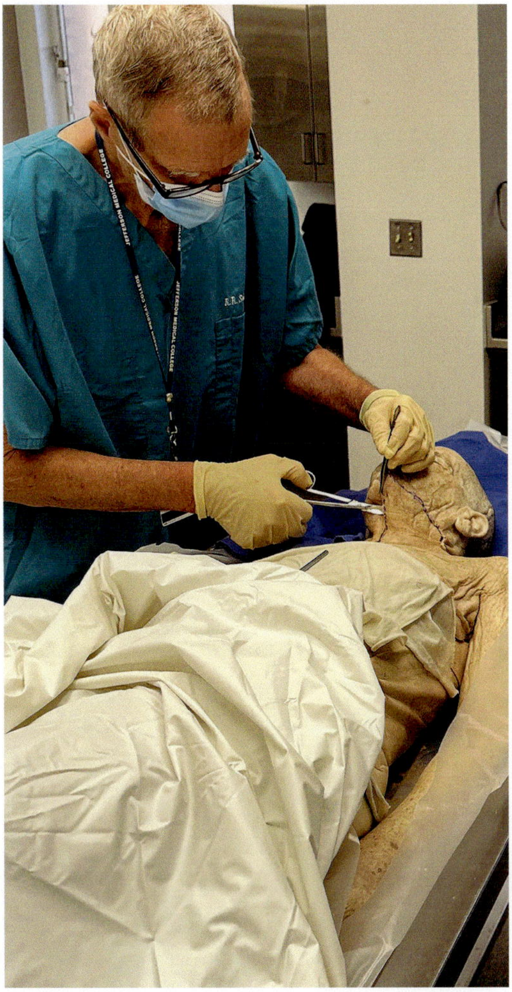

Fig. 1.4 Dr. Schmidt with prepared and embalmed cadaver

Further Reading

Ashraf Aziz M, McKenzie JC, Wilson JS, Cowie RJ, Ayeni SA, Dunn BK. The human cadaver in the age of biomedical informatics. Anat Rec. 2002;269:20–32.

Brenner E. Human body preservation—old and new techniques. J Anat. 2014:316–44.

Mayer RG. Embalming history, theory and practice. 4th ed. New York: McGraw Hill; 2006. p. 457–98.

Shrestha S, Bhattarai S, Mahat S, Jha M, Amgain K. Embalming: history to its recent advancements. Europasian J Med Sci. 2019;1(1):62–8.

2 The Forehead and Brow

Edward H. Bedrossian Jr., Sathyadeepak Ramesh, Bradley N. Lemke, Alison H. Watson, and Richard R. Schmidt

Introduction

In this chapter, the anatomy of the forehead and brow will be studied first by dissection in a direct layer-by-layer approach, starting superficially at the skin and proceeding to the periosteum. Anatomic study is continued, in another cadaver, using a small incisional endoscopic forehead technique, which is then converted to a bi-coronal forehead flap.

The approach to forehead and brow lifting first and foremost involves a thorough understanding of the anatomy, terminology, and danger zones. The following anatomic review will assist with the dissection.

The soft tissue of the SCALP is traditionally divided into five layers (Fig. 2.1). Superficial to deep these include: (1) the skin, (2) subcutaneous tissue, (3) galea aponeurosis (which is continuous with the SMAS, and splits to encompass the frontalis muscle), (4) loose areolar tissue, and (5) the periosteum of the frontal bone.

> **Clinical Correlation**
> Surgery to address forehead and brow aging lifts these layers as a composite with endoscopic and coronal brow lift procedures, but in the subcutaneous plane with pretrichial, mid-forehead, or supraciliary eyebrow lift procedures.

Richard R. Schmidt has died before the publication of this book.

E. H. Bedrossian Jr., MD, FACS (✉)
Wills Eye Hospital, Sydney Kimmel Medical College of Thomas Jefferson University, Philadelphia, PA, USA

Oculo-Facial Plastics Department, Wills Eye Hospital, Philadelphia, PA, USA

Clinical Professor Ophthalmology, Oculofacial Plastic Orbital Reconstructive Surgery, Lewis Katz School of Medicine at Temple University, Philadelphia, PA, USA

S. Ramesh, MD
The Center for Eye and Facial Plastic Surgery, Somerset, NJ, USA
e-mail: info@deepakrameshmd.com

B. N. Lemke, MD, FACS
Lemke Facial Surgery, Madison, WI, USA

Department of Ophthalmology and Visual Sciences, School of Medicine and Public Health, University of Wisconsin-Madison, Madison, WI, USA
e-mail: lemke@lemkefacialsurgery.com

A. H. Watson, MD, FACS
Department of Oculoplastic and Orbital Surgery, Wills Eye Hospital, Philadelphia, PA, USA
e-mail: awatson@willseye.org

R. R. Schmidt, PhD (Deceased)
Department of Pathology, Anatomy and Cell Biology, Sydney Kimmel Medical College of Thomas Jefferson University, Philadelphia, PA, USA

E. H. Bedrossian Jr et al. (eds.), *Anatomy of the Forehead, Face, and Neck*,
https://doi.org/10.1007/978-3-031-56140-5_2

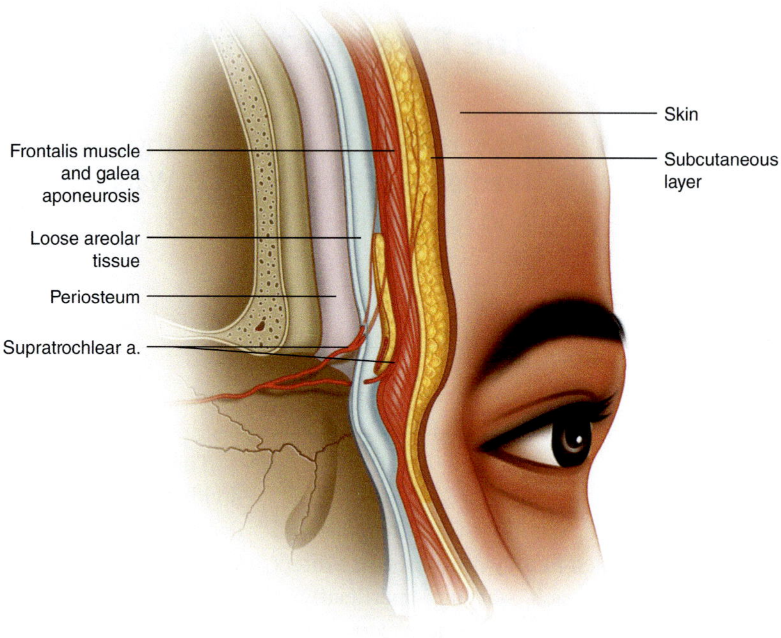

Fig. 2.1 Layers of the scalp

Forehead anatomy is simple, but the terminology is confusing as there is more than one name for the same structure. It becomes more complex near the superior orbital rim and zygomatic arch (Fig. 2.2). In the temporal area, there are two important layers:

The Superficial Temporalis Fascia (STF)

STF is also known as the temporoparietal fascia. It is continuous with the galea aponeurotica superiorly, as well as the superficial musculoaponeurotic system (SMAS) inferiorly (see Chap. 3). The forehead neurovasculature, and in particular the superficial temporal artery and the frontal branch of the facial nerve both travel within this layer.

Clinical Correlations

The superficial temporal artery lies more superficially inside the multilaminar tissue of the STF, while the frontal branch of the facial nerve lies on the posterior surface of this layer. Dissection deep to the superficial temporalis fascia adds protection to the facial nerve.

The superficial temporalis fascia can serve as donor tissue for reconstructive surgery.

The Deep Temporalis Fascia (DTF)

DTF is also known as the intermediate fascia and innominate fascia. It directly overlies and envelops the temporalis muscle. At the level of

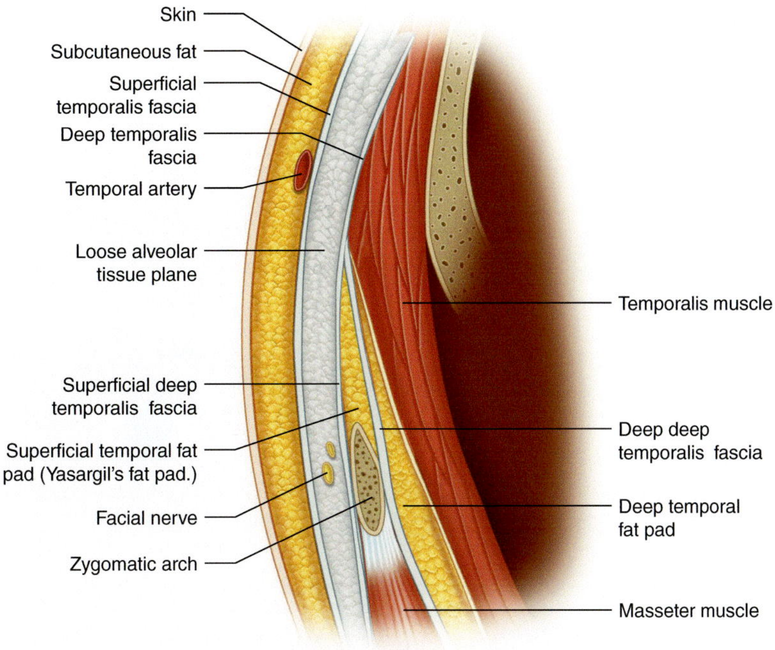

Fig. 2.2 Layers at the temporal area

the superior orbital rim, the anatomy then becomes more complicated as the DTF itself splits into a superficial (superficial deep temporalis fascia) and a deep layer (deep deep temporalis fascia), enveloping the superficial temporal fat pad (Yasargil's fat pad) before inserting onto the superior aspect of the zygomatic arch.

Therefore, below the level of the superior orbital rim, there are actually three fascial layers—the superficial temporal fascia, the superficial layer of the deep temporal fascia, and the deep layer of the deep temporal fascia.

The Temporal Line of Fusion (TLF)

TLF is also known as the superior temporal line (STL). It represents the location where the two layers (superficial temporalis fascia and the deep temporalis fascia) fuse together, then attach to the periosteum (Fig. 2.3). This fusion is known as the conjoint tendon. The line separates the temporal fossa zone from the central forehead zone anteriorly and the calvarium posteriorly. It marks the site of origin of the temporalis muscle.

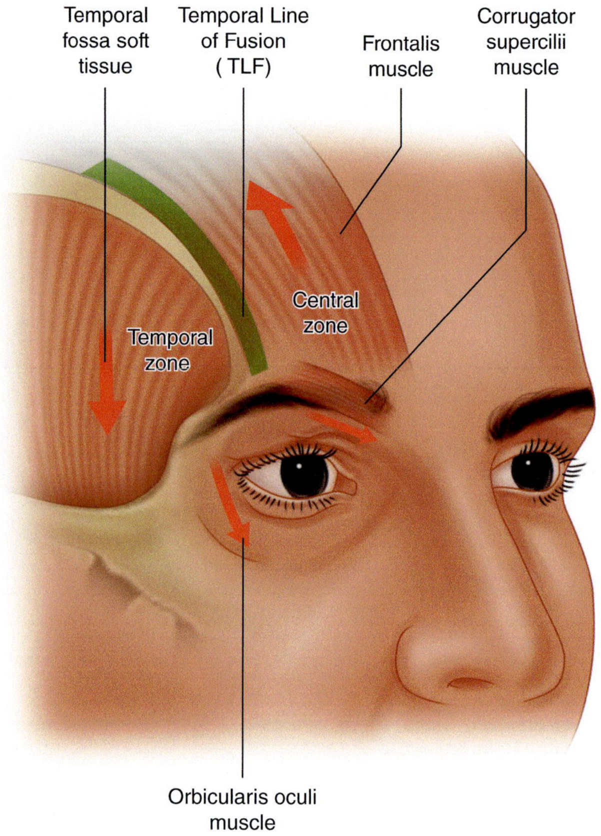

Fig. 2.3 Temporal line of fusion separating the "temporal zone" from "central zone"

Brow and Hemi Forehead Dissection

Skin Incisions

1. For the purpose of this dissection, with a #10 or 15 blade create a *hemicoronal* incision, starting from the inferior border of the tragus to the midline of the forehead (Fig. 2.4a).
2. Carry the incision from the midline to the glabella (Fig. 2.4b).

Subcutaneous Dissection

1. Dissect sharply in the subcutaneous plane to separate the skin and adherent subcutaneous fat layer from the underlying galea aponeurotica/frontalis muscle (Figs. 2.5 and 2.6).
2. Reflect the skin and subcutaneous fat layer inferiorly, toward the inferior orbital rim. Note the vertically oriented sensory nerves (Fig. 2.7) which are branches of the first division of the trigeminal nerve (CN V), stemming from the supraorbital and supratrochlear bundles (Fig. 2.8).
3. Note that the underlying frontalis muscle is a vertically oriented muscle (Fig. 2.9). It is a paired muscle which originates from and is encased by the galea aponeurotica.
4. Continue the subcutaneous dissection inferiorly to the brow and note how the frontalis muscle fibers also inserts into the dermis posterior to the brow (Fig. 2.10).

   Subcutaneous undermining safely separates the skin from the SMAS layer. In the forehead and glabella, the SMAS contains the frontalis and procerus muscles with the arteries passing superficially on the muscles and the nerves rising on the posterior muscle surface, more deeply within the SMAS.
5. Continue the dissection inferior to the brow and note how frontalis fibers interdigitate

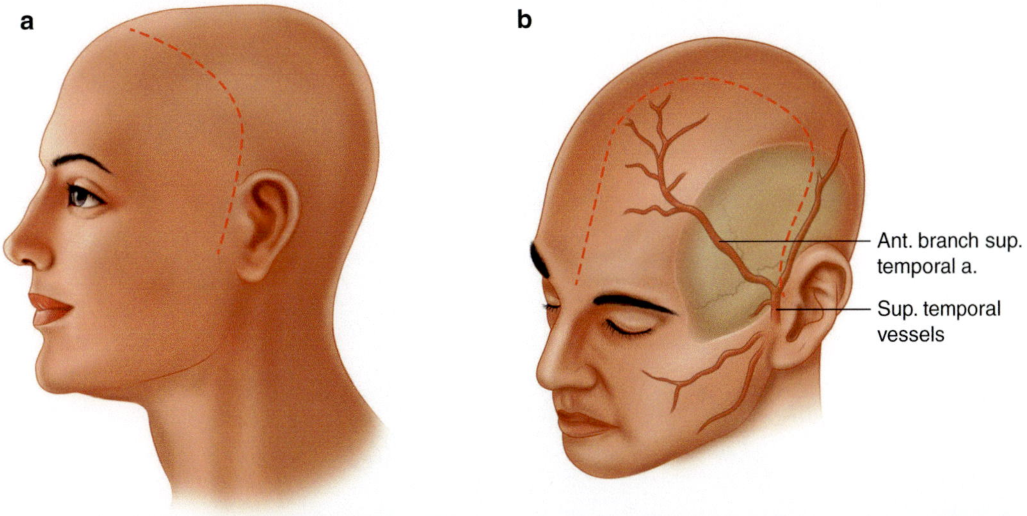

Fig. 2.4 Hemicoronal incision, from inferior border of tragus to the midline of forehead (**a**), then to the glabella (**b**)

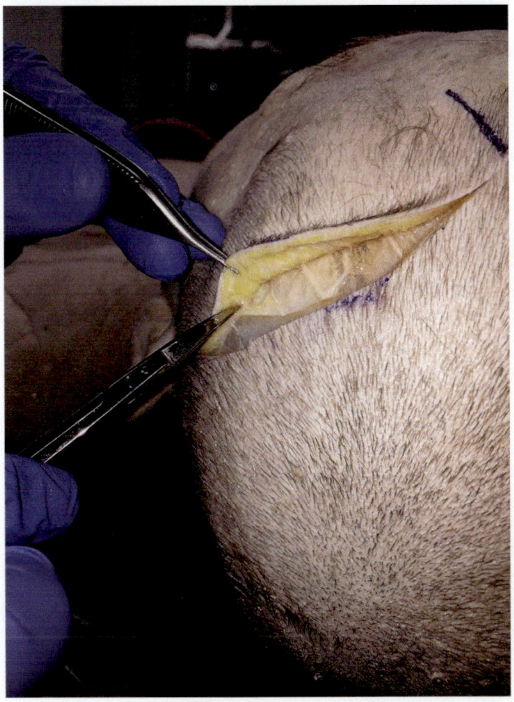

Fig. 2.5 Initial skin incision and subcutaneous plane between skin/subcutaneous fat layer and the underlying galea aponeurotica and frontalis muscle

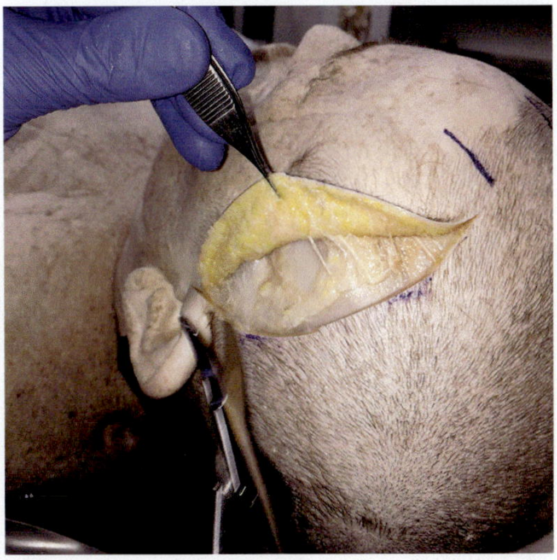

Fig. 2.6 Extended subcutaneous dissection exposing underlying galea aponeurotiia/frontalis muscle

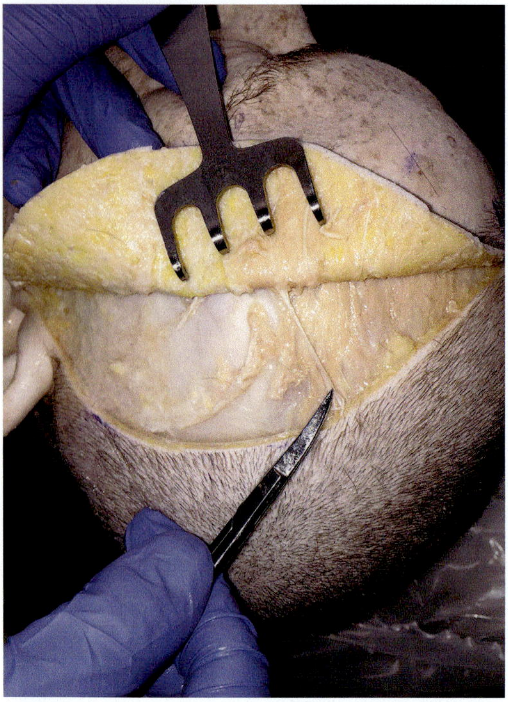

Fig. 2.7 Vertically oriented sensory nerve (CNV 1)

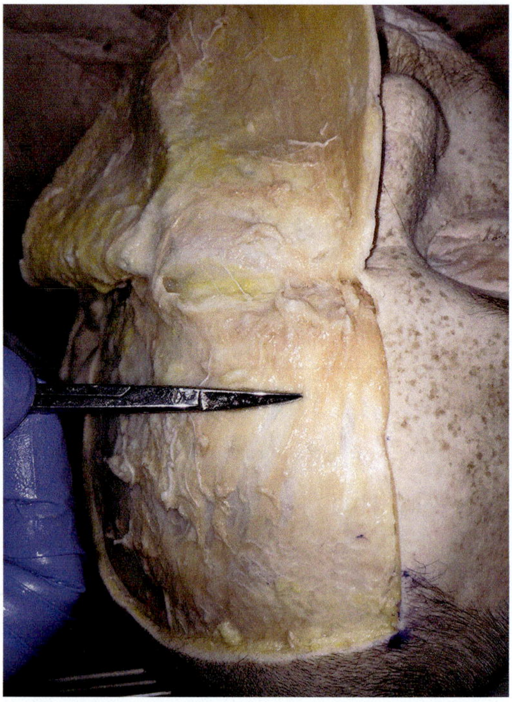

Fig. 2.8 Supraorbital and supratrochlear nerve bundles

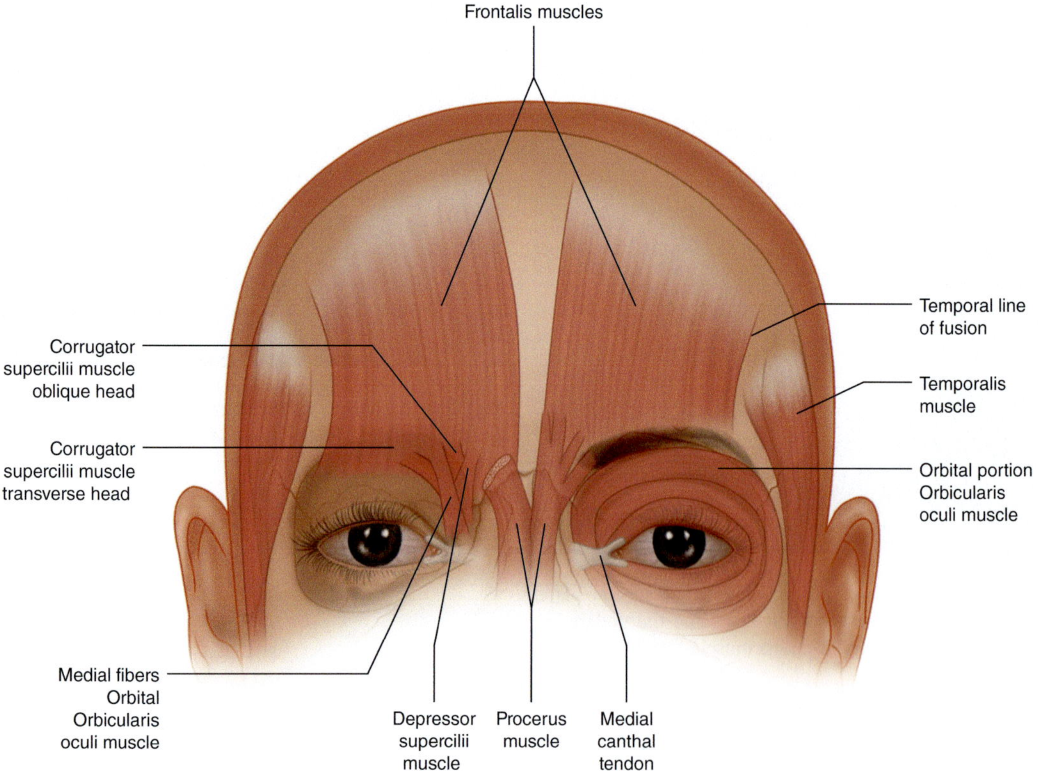

Fig. 2.9 Forehead and eyebrow muscles. Note the vertically oriented frontalis muscle and brow depressors (procerus, corrugator supercilii, depressor supercilii, and medial portion orbicularis oculi muscles)

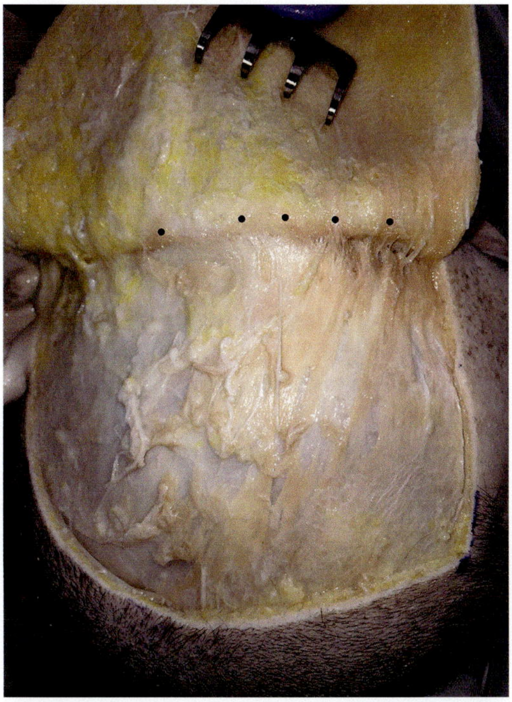

Fig. 2.10 Frontalis muscle extending into the dermis (black dots) posterior to the brow

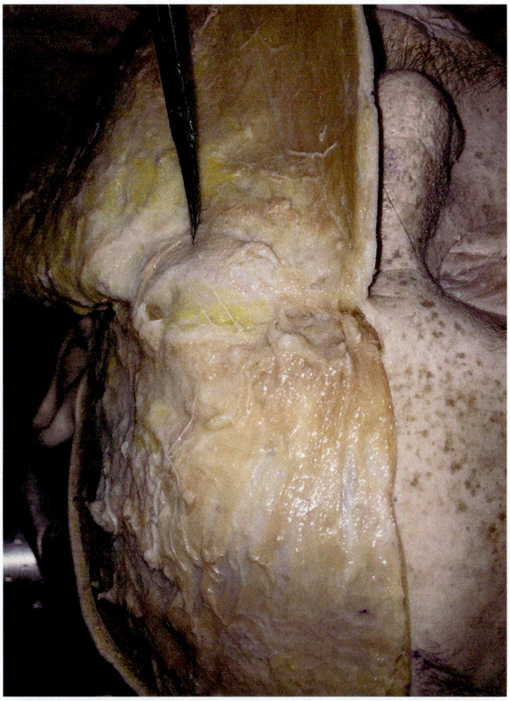

Fig. 2.11 Orbital orbicularis muscle (pointer) in reflected skin flap

with the orbital portion of the orbicularis oculi muscle (Fig. 2.11) and centrally with the procerus muscle in the glabellar region.

Clinical Correlations

The frontalis muscle raises the eyebrow creating the horizontal rhytids evident in the mid-forehead.

Subcutaneous undermining with skin excision provides forehead lifting options. Incisions can be camouflaged in the eyebrow (Fig. 2.12), along hairline (Fig. 2.13) or be made in prominent forehead creases (Fig. 2.14).

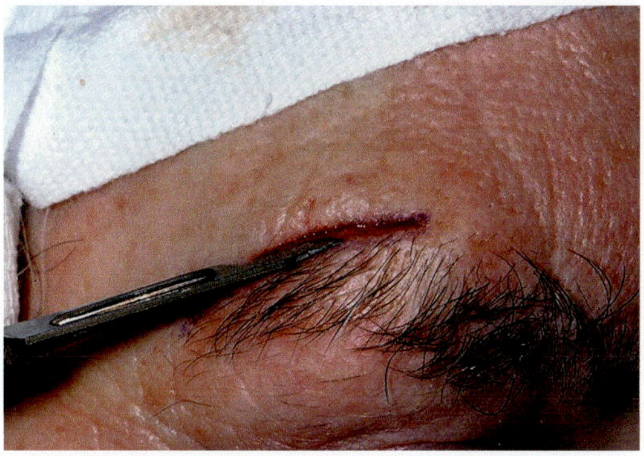

Fig. 2.12 Supraciliary brow lift. Note the angle of the scalpel to parallel the hair follicles

6. Continue the subcutaneous dissection inferiorly to the inferior edge of the zygomatic arch.
7. Continue the subcutaneous dissection into the glabella, exposing the underlying procerus muscle and corrugator supercilii muscles (Fig. 2.9). See Forehead Myotomy Muscle Stripping below (Figs. 2.46, 2.47, 2.48, 2.49, 2.50 and 2.51).

Frontalis Muscle and Galea Aponeurotica

1. Next incise the *frontalis muscle* following the hemicoronal skin incision laterally along temporal line of fusion, and then along the midline to the supra orbital rim (Fig. 2.15).
2. Reflect the frontalis muscle and galea aponeurotica anteriorly (Fig. 2.16).
3. Note how the galea aponeurotica is present on both the anterior and posterior surfaces of the frontalis muscle.
4. Note how the frontalis muscle laterally extends to terminate just medial to the superior temporal line of fusion at the location of the conjoint tendon where the periosteum and galea are tightly adherent.

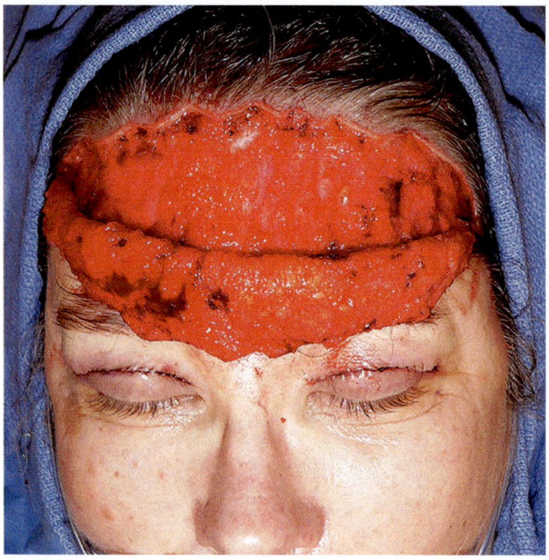

Fig. 2.13 Pretrichial brow lift with subcutaneous dissection

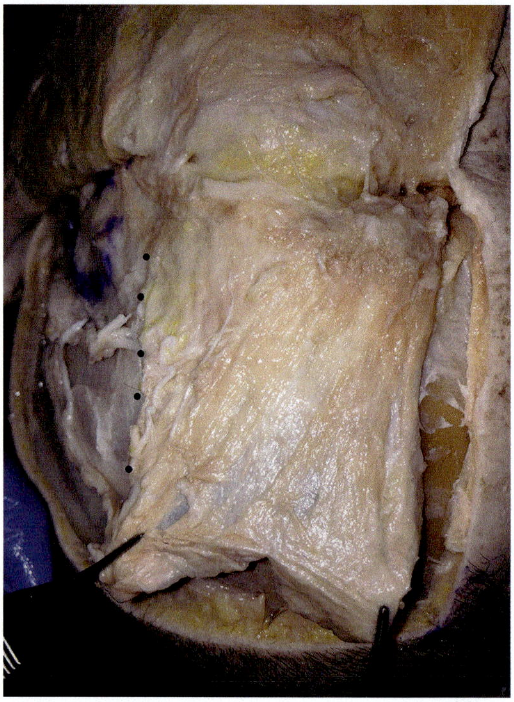

Fig. 2.15 Incision site of frontalis muscle laterally (dots) and in the midline

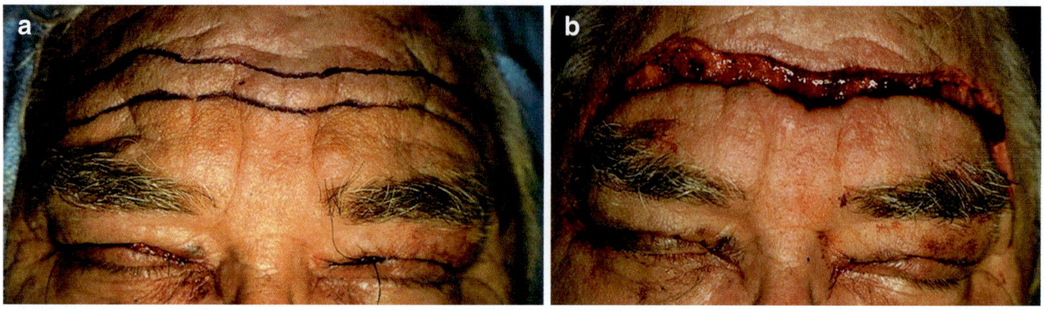

Fig. 2.14 Mid forehead skin marking in deep forehead creases (**a**) and skin excision (**b**)

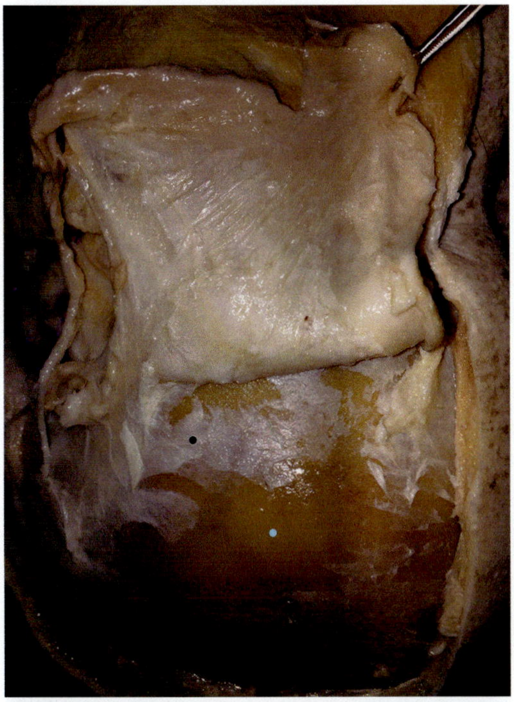

Fig. 2.16 Reflected frontalis muscle flap exposing shiny galea aponeuotica. Note periosteum (black dot) and frontal bone (blue dot)

Clinical Correlations

At the time of brow and forehead lifting surgery, the temporal zone and central zone are "joined" by lysing the conjoint tendon from the temporal line of fusion.

Temporally, the galea aponeurotic continues as the superficial temporalis fascia. Inferiorly, in the mid and lower face (see Chap. 3), it continues with the superficial musculoaponeurotic system (SMAS), which then proceeds to the platysma in the neck (see Chap. 4 and Fig. 4.14).

The motor function innervation to the frontalis is by the frontal branch of the seventh cranial nerve, explaining why brow ptosis is seen in Bell's palsy and other seventh nerve palsies.

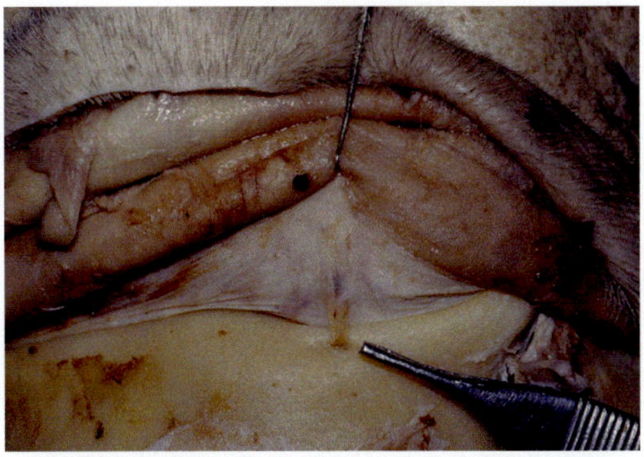

Fig. 2.17 Superior orbital rim, with supraorbital nerve emerging from supraorbital foramen

Periosteum and Frontal Bone

1. Once the frontalis muscle and the galea aponeurotica are reflected anteriorly, identify the *periosteum* (Fig. 2.16) of the frontal bone. When this last layer (periosteum) is incised, the bare surface of the frontal bone is visible (Fig. 2.16).
2. Proceed inferiorly until the superior orbital rim is visualized. One or multiple foramina (Fig. 2.17) or notches will be visualized medially, with neurovascular structures emerging from the orbit and traveling superiorly.

Clinical Correlation

Sensation to the forehead and brow is primarily supplied by the ophthalmic division of the trigeminal nerve, namely from its supraorbital and supratrochlear branches. The supraorbital nerve emerges from its named foramen at or just above the superior orbital rim (Fig. 2.17). This is the location for a supraorbital nerve block of local anesthesia.

3. Trace how it divides into a medial superficial division and deep lateral division that may rarely exit from separate foramina.
4. Identify the supratrochlear nerve supply as it proceeds to the medial forehead.

Clinical Correlation
Care is taken with direct endoscopic visualization by the brow lift surgeon, to preserve these nerves, while carefully releasing the adjacent periosteum to permit elevation of the brow (see section "Complete the Central and Nasal Brow Release" below).

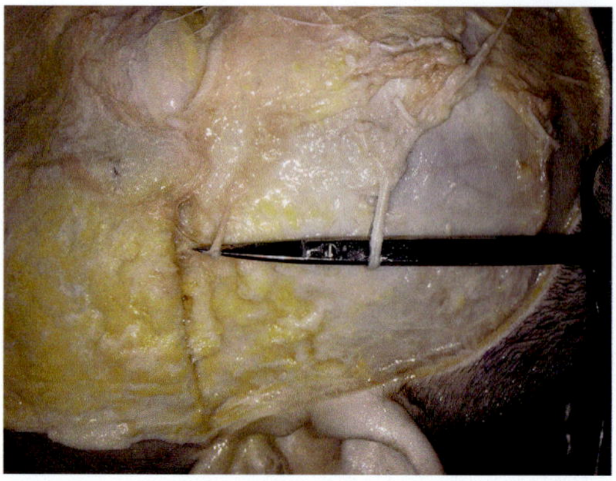

Fig. 2.19 Superficial temporal artery (body of scissors) and facial nerve (tip of scissors)

Temporal Dissection

1. Identify the conjoint tendon at the temporal fusion line (Fig. 2.18). It is the origin of the temporalis muscle and marks the boundary between the temple (temporal zone) and the forehead (central zone).
2. Identify the superficial temporal artery, deep to the skin but in the superficial layer of the multi-lamella of the superficial temporalis fascia (Fig. 2.19).

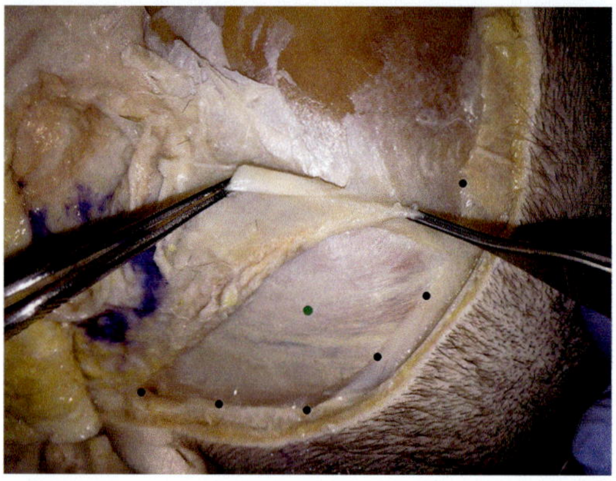

Fig. 2.20 Superficial Temporal Fascia (STF) in forceps. Note the site of the STF incision (black dots) and the underlying. Deep Temporal Fascial DTF (green dot)

Clinical Correlation
Knowledge of this superficial anatomy is appreciated at the time of temporal artery biopsy.

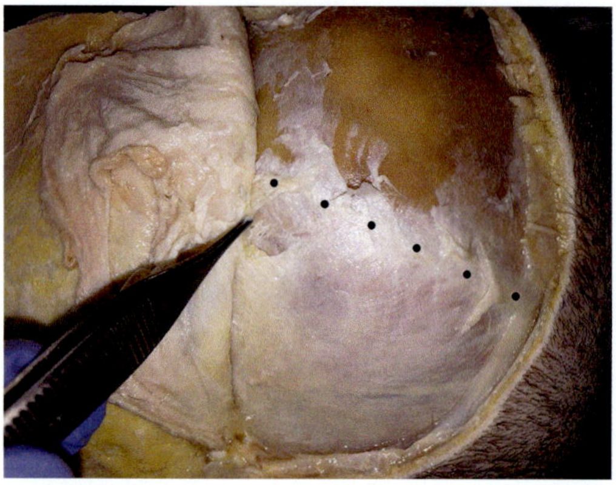

Fig. 2.18 Conjoint tendon (black dots)

3. Incise the superficial temporalis fascia (Fig. 2.20) widely, starting at the initial skin incision.
4. Identify the deep temporalis fascia as the glistening layer overlying the temporalis muscle (Fig. 2.20).
5. Bluntly dissect underneath the superficial temporalis fascia, just on the surface of the deep temporalis fascia (Fig. 2.21), in the loose areolar tissue plane by elevating the superficial temporalis fascia with forceps and periosteal elevator.
6. Continue the incision of the superficial temporalis fascia following the arc of the origin of the temporalis muscle along the temporal line of fusion (conjoint tendon) (Fig. 2.22).

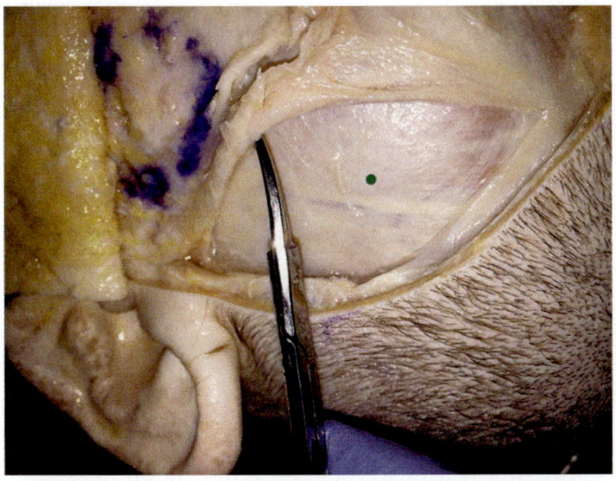

Fig. 2.21. Scissors between STF and DTF (green dot). Note Yassergil's fat pad (purple circle) also called the superficial temporal fat pad seen through the superficial temporal fascia. It marks the area where the facial nerve crosses the zygomatic arch

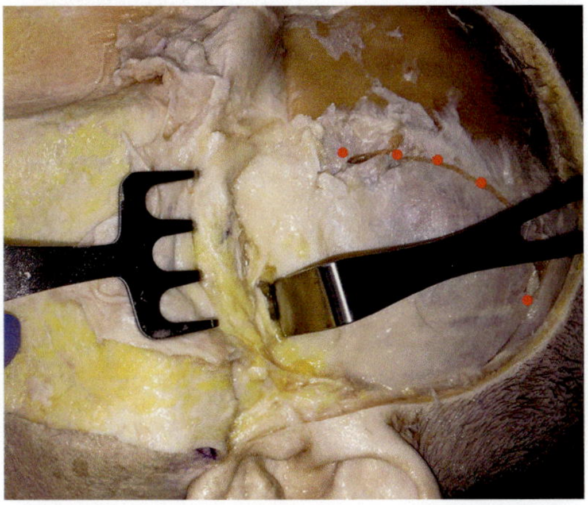

Fig. 2.22 Incision site of the superficial temporal fascia along conjoint tendon (red dots)

7. Proceed with the blunt dissection between the superficial temporal fascia and the deep temporal fascia, inferiorly to the level of the lateral canthal tendon and until the zygomatic arch is reached (Fig. 2.23).

Clinical Correlation

An elevator (e.g., Kilner or Bristow) is introduced between the superficial temporalis fascia and deep temporalis fascia for a closed Gillies' approach for reduction of an isolated zygomatic arch fracture (Fig. 2.24).

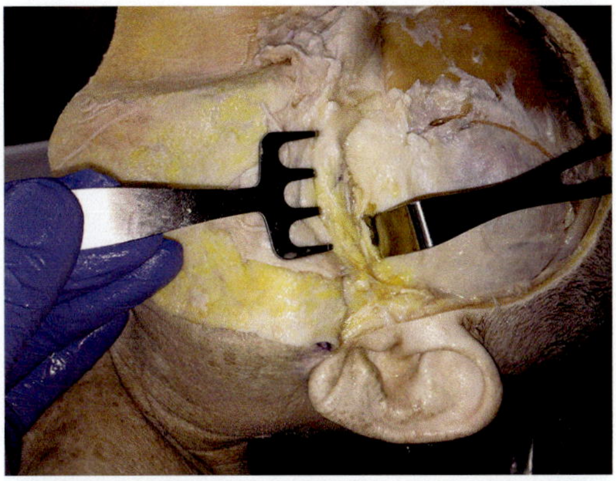

Fig. 2.23 Superficial temporal fascia reflected in rake, retractor below zygomatic arch

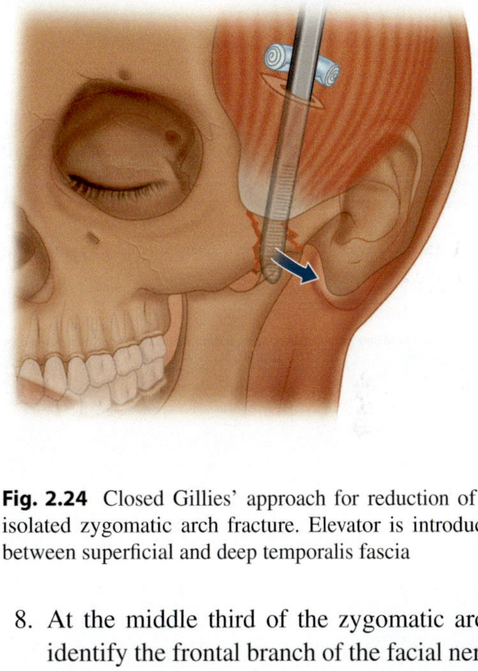

Fig. 2.24 Closed Gillies' approach for reduction of an isolated zygomatic arch fracture. Elevator is introduced between superficial and deep temporalis fascia

8. At the middle third of the zygomatic arch, identify the frontal branch of the facial nerve seen emerging just over the periosteum (Fig. 2.25) and crossing the zygomatic arch to travel just on the surface of the superficial temporalis fascia.
9. Note the accuracy of its relationship to Pitanguy's line drawn on the skin extending from near the tragus of the ear to the lateral aspect of the eyebrow (Fig. 2.26).

Clinical Correlation
Understanding the relationships between these planes and the frontal branch of the facial nerve is critical. Superior to the zygomatic arch, surgical dissection must proceed *deep* to the superficial temporalis fascia to avoid injuring the facial nerve.

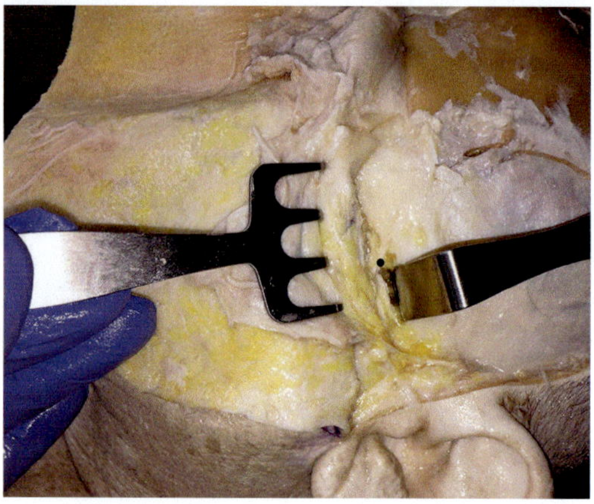

Fig. 2.25 Exposed facial nerve (black dot) crossing the zygomatic arch

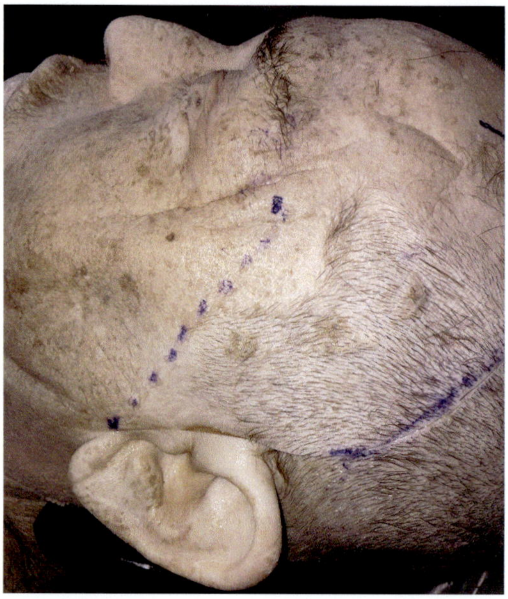

Fig. 2.26 Pitanguy line: drawn from near the tragus to the lateral aspect of brow marking where facial nerve crosses the zygomatic arch

10. Identify Yasargil's Fat Pad (Fig. 2.27). Also called the superficial temporal fat pad, it lies between the deep and superficial layers of the deep temporalis fascia which divides about 2.5 cm above the zygomatic arch (Fig. 2.2).

Clinical Correlation
Maintaining temporal dissection in the plane of the superficial temporal fat will prevent injury to the overlying facial nerve.

11. Identify the medial zygomaticotemporal vein, also called the Sentinel vein (Figs. 2.27 and 2.28).

Clinical Correlation
The sentinel vein is an essential indicator to proximity to the frontal branch of the facial nerve during temporal dissection at the time of brow lifting. It traverses the deep plane of dissection to enter the superficial temporalis fascia adjacent to the facial nerve. Cautery of the vessel intraoperatively could injure the frontal branch of the facial nerve.

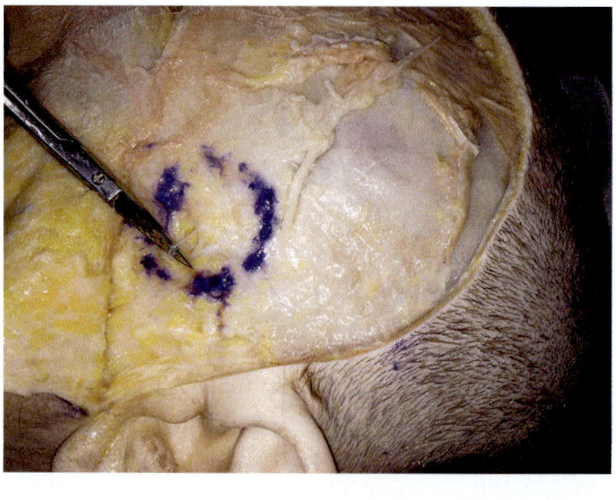

Fig. 2.27 Yasargil's fat pad is seen through the superficial temporalis fascia and the superficial layers of the deep temporalis fascia. Note the facial nerve above the scissors and the sentinel vein under the scissor tips

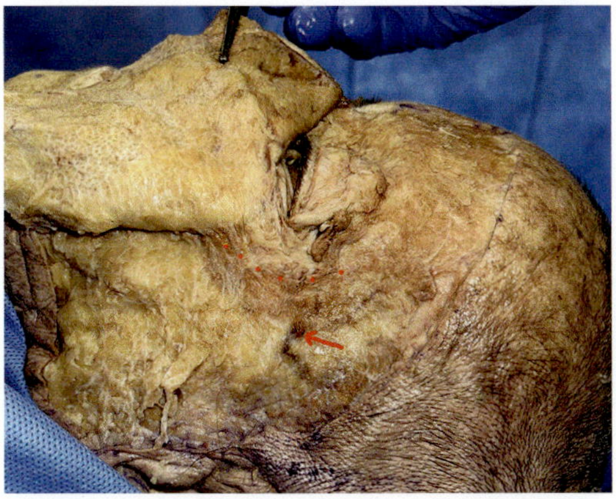

Fig. 2.28 The sentinel vein (arrow) in another specimen. The skin and subcutaneous flap is reflected medially in forceps, exposing the orbital portion of the orbicularis muscle at the lateral orbital rim (red dots)

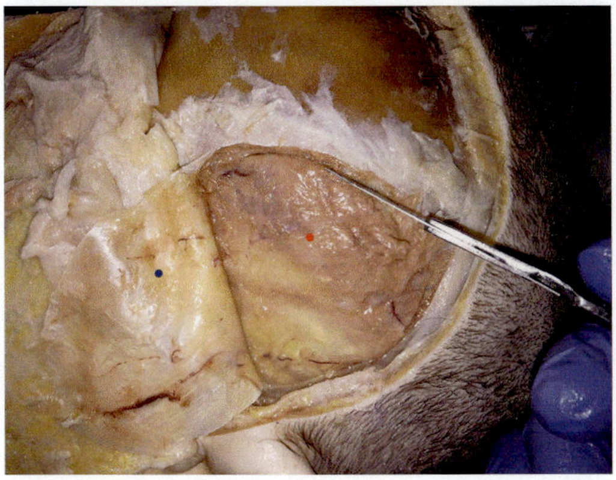

Fig. 2.29 The deep temporalis fascia (blue dot), superficial to the temporalis muscle, was incised along the temporal line of fusion and reflected over the zygomatic arch exposing the temporalis muscle (red dot). Note the deeper incision of the temporalis muscle (blade) along temporal line of fusion

12. Incise the deep temporalis fascia and visualize the body of the temporalis muscle.
13. Incise the temporalis muscle along the temporal line of fusion (Fig. 2.29).
14. Reflect the temporalis muscle anteriorly (Fig. 2.30). Note that it exposes the temporal fossa.
15. On the undersurface of this muscle will be multiple perforating deep temporal nerves and vessel (zygomaticotemporal vein) (Fig. 2.31).

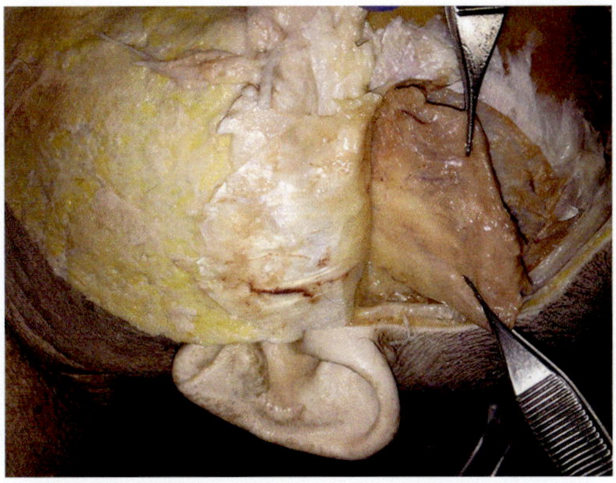

Fig. 2.30 Temporalis muscle flap

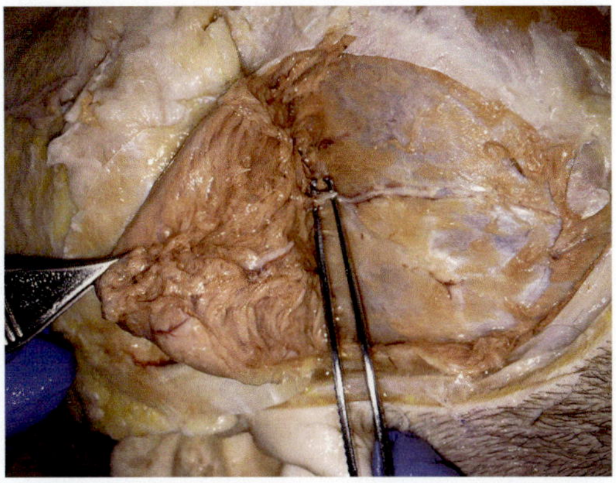

Fig. 2.31 Deep sentinel vein (medial zygomaticotemporal vein) on undersurface of the reflected temporalis muscle

16. Follow the temporalis muscle itself as it travels inferiorly, deep to the zygomatic arch, to attach to the coronoid process of the mandible.
17. Deep to the temporalis muscle, identify the periosteum and bone of the temporal fossa. This concludes the layered approach to the anatomy of the brow and forehead.

Brow and Forehead Dissection: Endoscopic Approach

In this section, the study of forehead and brow anatomy will require another cadaver. A major portion of small incision endoscopic brow or forehead lift surgery does not require an endoscope. Section "Brow and Hemi Forehead Dissection" above provides a strong foundation in forehead and brow anatomy. What follows is an anatomic exercise demonstrating a step-by-step approach to an endoscopic brow and forehead lift for those steps not requiring an endoscope. Those steps include (1) scalp and temporal incision placement, (2) subperiosteal dissection of the posterior zone, (3) subperiosteal dissection of the central zone, (4) dissection in the temporal zone, and (5) connection from the temporal zone into the central zone. Many surgeons prefer using an endoscope for this last step.

Since endoscopes are not standard equipment found in the cadaver laboratory, those steps requiring an endoscope will be described with illustrations. Those steps include (1) endoscopic dissection at orbital rim, (2) release of tissue at the arcus marginalis, (3) release of glabellar musculature, and for some surgeons, (4) connection from the temporal zone into the central zone.

Also described are bone fixation techniques. For those interested, an endoscopic brow surgery course is advised to better appreciate the use of the endoscope and orientation through the endoscope.

Finally, the small incisions are converted to a bi-coronal forehead flap.

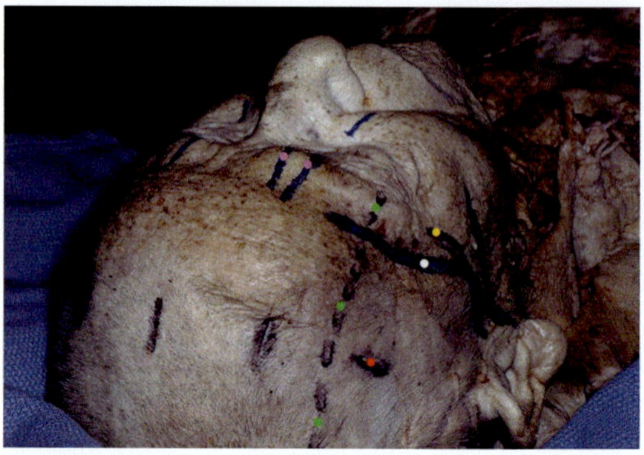

Fig. 2.32 Markings for endoscopic incisions. Note the temporal incision marking (red dot), site of the temporal line of fusion (green dots), Zygomatic arch (yellow dot), suprorbital and supratrochlear neurovascular bundles (pink dots) and Pitanguy's line (white dot)

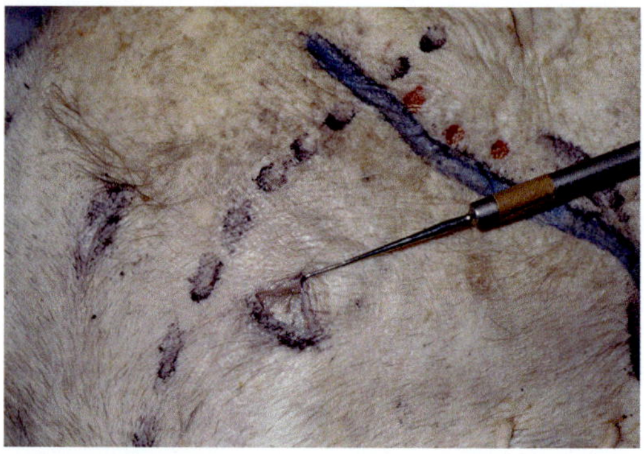

Fig. 2.33 Temporal incision thru skin and subcutaneous layer

Skin Incisions

1. For the purpose of this dissection *mark five incisions*, three on the scalp and two temporally (Fig. 2.32).
2. The *central scalp incision* is 2 cm long, radially oriented and placed in the midline just behind the anterior hair line.
3. The *two lateral or paracentral scalp* incisions are also 2 cm long, radially oriented and alien with the lateral canthus, posterior to the hairline, just medial to the superior temporal line.
4. For the three scalp incisions (one central and two paracentral), use a #10 or #15 blade to cut through all scalp layers down to the periosteum.
5. As the incisions are made, identify the five layers of the scalp: (1) the skin, (2) subcutaneous tissue, (3) galea aponeurosis, (4) loose areolar tissue, and (5) periosteum.
6. The *two temporal incisions*, one each on the right and on the left, are 3 cm long, oriented in the coronal plane, posterior to the hairline. The incisions are made in an elliptical manner.
7. Use a #15 blade to incise through the skin and subcutaneous layer along the ellipse (Fig. 2.33).
8. Manually elevate the lateral brow in the location of the designed temporal incision to confirm optimal vector lift for the desired temporal brow contour.

Dissection Zones

There are three brow lift dissection zones: (1) posterior (vertex), (2) frontal or central and (3) temporal (Fig. 2.34). The plane of dissection in the posterior and central zones are subperiosteal. However, each temporal dissection occurs in a plane deep to the superficial temporalis fascial but superficial to the deep temporalis fascia.

Vertex and Posterior Scalp Dissection

Use the central and two paracentral incisions to perform subperiosteal dissection posteriorly (Fig. 2.35) with a parietal periosteal elevator, to the vertex and toward the occiput.

Central Dissection: Forehead

Use the central and two paracentral scalp incisions to anteriorly perform subperiosteal forehead dissection (Fig. 2.36) with a half-curved forehead elevator or periosteal elevator, toward the superior orbital rim and the dorsum of the nose. This can be done completely by feel, without an endoscope, to a level about 1.5 cm above the superior orbital rim.

> **Clinical Correlation**
> During endoscopic brow lift, nasally this release will require direct endoscopic visualization to avoid inadvertent injury to the supraorbital and supratrochlear nerves (as below).

Dissect to the conjoint tendon at the temporal line of fusion, which is the lateral boundary of this central dissection zone.

Temporal Dissection

1. Through each 3 cm temporal incision (Fig. 2.37) dissect inferiorly through the superficial temporalis fascia with a straight frontotemporal dissector or periosteal elevator

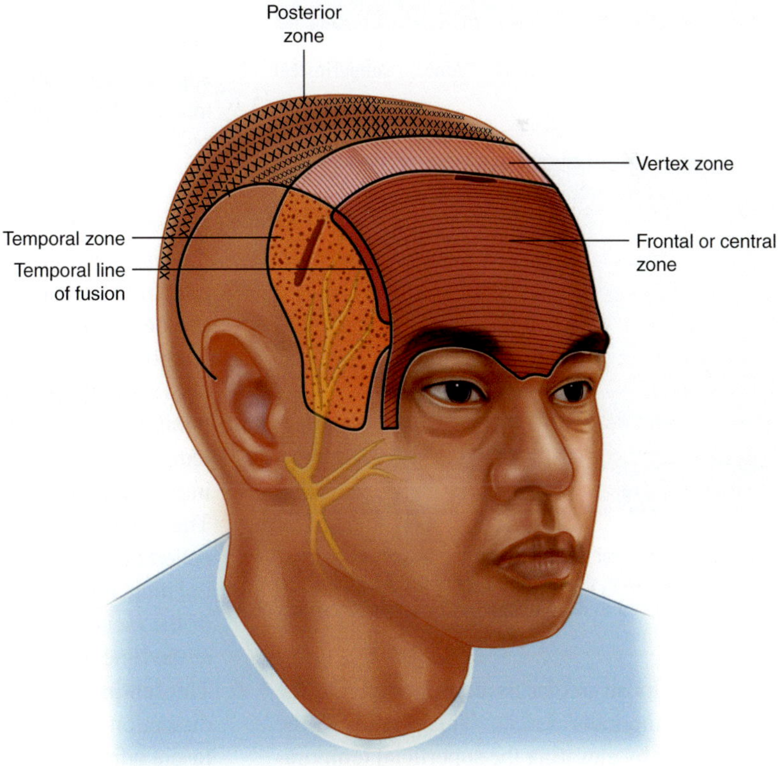

Fig. 2.34 Endoscopic dissection zones

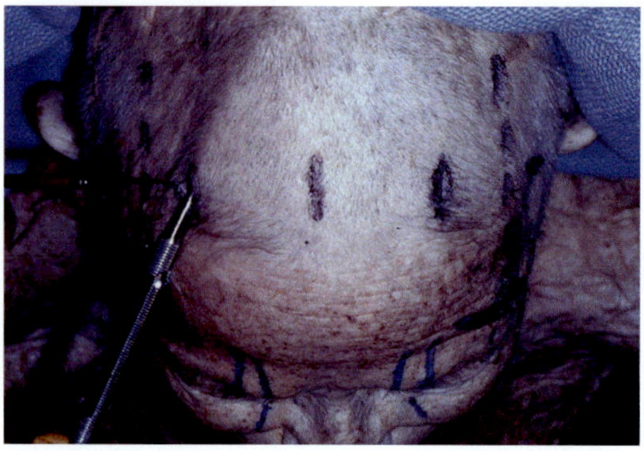

Fig. 2.35 Posterior (vertex) zone, subperiosteal dissection

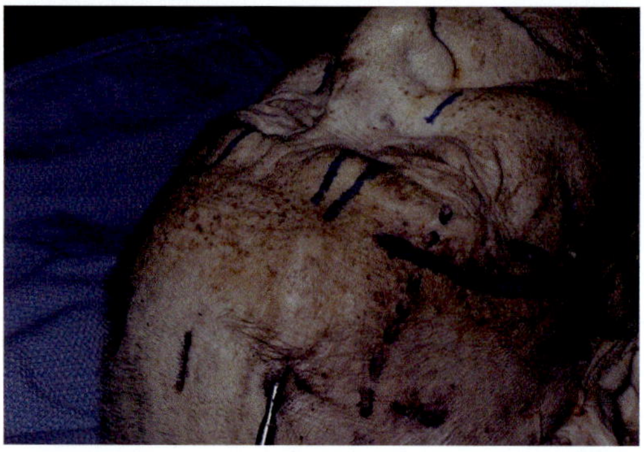

Fig. 2.36 Central forehead zone, subperiosteal dissection

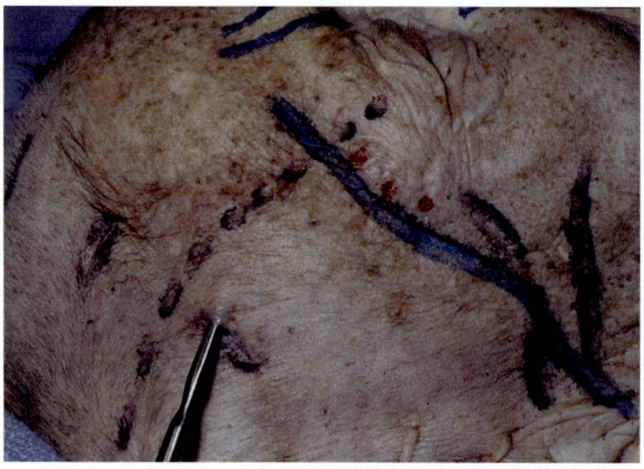

Fig. 2.37 Temporal zone dissection: dissector in loose areolar tissue plane, deep to the superficial temporal fascia, but superficial to deep temporal fascia near the superior temporal line

into the loose areolar tissue, superficial to the deep temporalis fascia. This can also be achieved by elevating the superficial temporalis fascia with forceps, then carefully incising the superficial temporalis fascia with a curved Steven's scissor.

2. Blunt dissection is then used in a spreading fashion to continue down to the deep temporalis fascia, which will be identified as the glistening layer overlying the temporalis muscle.

Clinical Correlation

Understanding the relationships between these planes and associated soft tissues is critical. As the frontal branch of the facial nerve is particularly vulnerable to injury with surgery in this region.

3. Continue dissection to the level of the lateral canthal tendon and medial one third of the zygomatic arch (Fig. 2.38). This is performed initially using direct visualization without the endoscope.

Clinical Correlation

It is in this plane that a Kilner or Bristow elevator is introduced for a closed Gillies' approach for reduction of an isolated zygomatic arch fracture (Fig. 2.24).

4. Introduce the endoscope and identify Yasergil's Fat Pad. Also called the superficial temporal fat pad (Fig. 2.27), it lies between the deep and superficial layers of the deep temporalis fascia which divides about 2.5 cm above the zygomatic arch. Maintaining temporal dissection in the plane of the superficial temporal fat will prevent injury to the overlying facial nerve.
5. The medial zygomaticotemporal vein, also called the sentinel vein (Fig. 2.39) is an essential indicator to proximity to the frontal branch of the facial nerve during temporal dissection at the time of brow lifting.
6. The sentinel vein traverses the deep plane of dissection to enter the superficial temporal fascia adjacent to the facial nerve. See if you can identify this vein in your dissection plane.

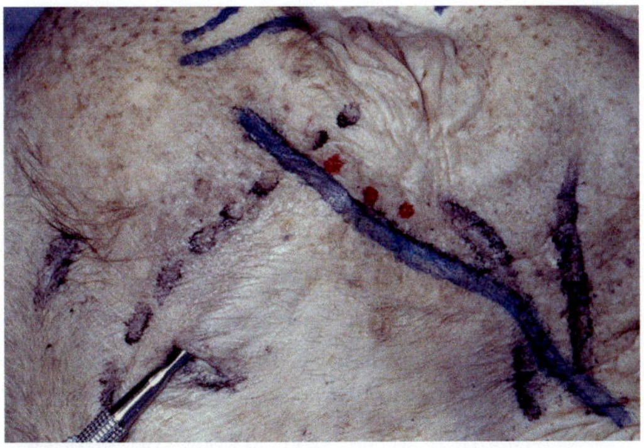

Fig. 2.38 Temporal zone dissection to level of lateral canthal tendon and zygomatic arch

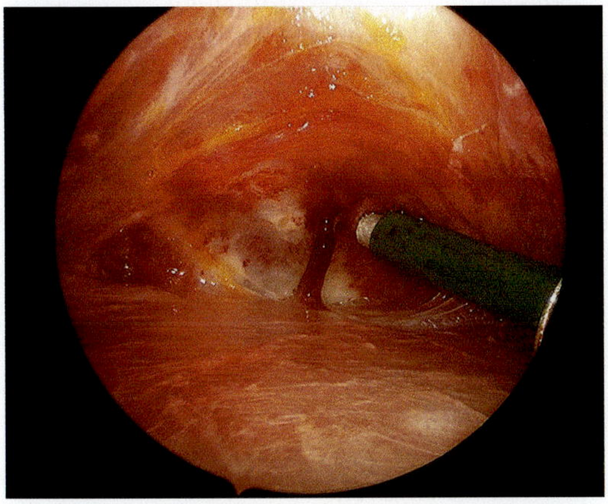

Fig. 2.39 Surgical endoscopic view of sentinel vein

Clinical Correlation
Cautery of the vessel intraoperatively could injure the frontal branch of the facial nerve.

7. Continue the temporal dissection and release the attachments along the medial third of the zygomatic arch.
8. Complete the temporal dissection anterosuperiorly (Fig. 2.38) toward the superior temporal line (conjoint tendon). Identify the conjoint tendon. It is a dense facial condensation of the superficial temporalis fascia and the deep temporalis fascia, which attaches to the skull at the superior temporal line.

Connection of the Temporal and Central Forehead Zones

To fully mobilize the forehead and brow, the forehead (central) and temporal zones must be connected at the level of the superior temporal lines (conjoint tendon) (Fig. 2.3).

1. Under direct endoscopic visualization or bimanually, identify the conjoint tendon.
2. Release it in a lateral (temporal zone) to medial (central zone) direction, as follows:
   (a) Place the straight frontotemporal dissector in the temporal incision.
   (b) Place the 30-degree endoscope or Freer elevator in the paracentral scalp incision.
   (c) Then dissect toward the central zone until the conjoint tendon is lysed at the superior temporal line, connecting the temporal and central zones (Fig 2.40).

Clinical Correlation
It is safest to use an endoscope for this step. Care is always taken to release the conjoint tendon, starting from the temporal zone moving toward the central zone, to avoid inadvertent injury to the facial nerve and sentinel vein.

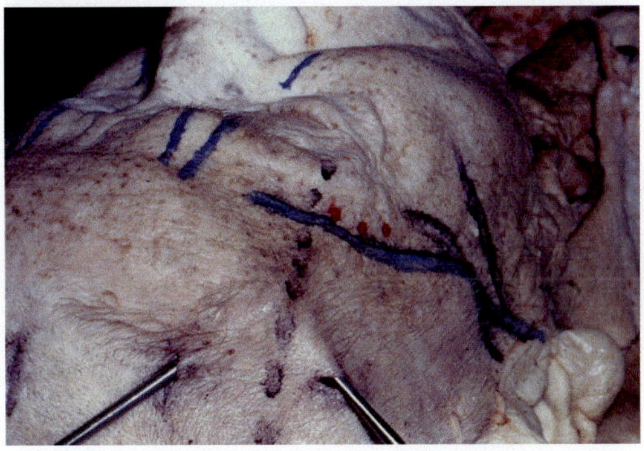

Fig. 2.40 Release at conjoint tendon. Left probe under periosteum, right probe through conjoint tendon

Complete the Central and Nasal Brow Release

1. Complete central release toward the lateral orbital rim (Fig. 2.41).
   (a) Place the endoscope in the central incision and the half-curved orbital rim dissector in the paracentral scalp incision (not shown).
   (b) Carry the dissection in the subperiosteal plane over the lateral orbital rim to the level of the lateral canthus with the curved orbital rim dissector.
2. Complete Central Release to expose the superior orbital rim.
   (a) With the endoscope through the temporal incision and the arcus marginalis dissector elevator through the lateral (paracentral) scalp incision, visualize the central zone toward the superior orbital rim (Fig. 2.42).
   (b) Dissect in the subperiosteal plane to the superior orbital rim. Using the sharp edge of the arcus marginalis dissector, ensure there is complete periosteal release along the superior orbital rim. Superior orbital fat may be exposed.
   (c) As you move nasally (Fig. 2.43) identify the trunks of the supraorbital (Fig. 2.44) and supratrochlear nerves as they emerge from their foramina.
   (d) Use a Metzenbaum scissors to spread parallel to the nerves to release the adjacent periosteum without nerve injury. The supratrochlear nerve innervates the medial forehead. The supraorbital nerve emerges from its named foramen at or just above the superior orbital rim.

Clinical and Anatomic Correlation
Sensation to the forehead and brow is primarily supplied by the ophthalmic division CN V, namely from its supraorbital and supratrochlear branches. Care is taken to preserve these nerves while carefully releasing the adjacent periosteum to permit elevation of the brow.

   (e) Identify nasal orbital fat in the roof of the orbit (Fig. 2.44). It may be difficult to find in the cadaver.

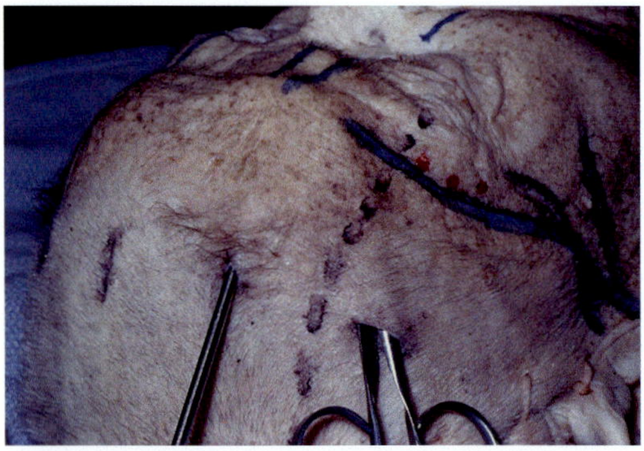

Fig. 2.41 Release of conjoint tendon toward superior orbital rim. Left probe under periosteum, scissors thru conjoint tendon

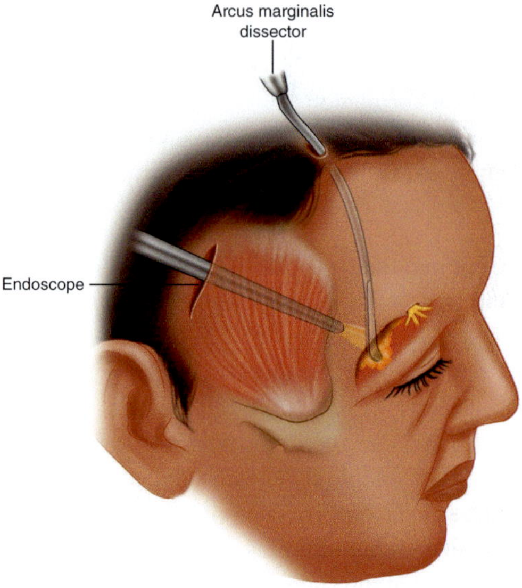

Fig. 2.42 Superior lateral orbital rim dissection

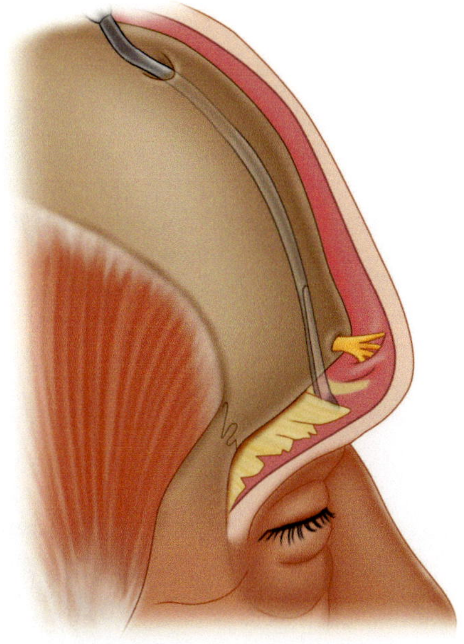

Fig. 2.43 Superior nasal orbital rim dissection toward neurovascular bundle

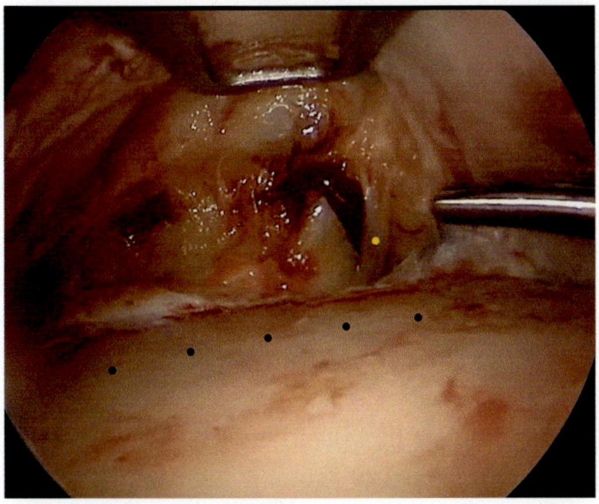

Fig. 2.44 Surgical endoscopic view of supraorbital nerve (yellow dot) at the supraorbital rim (black dots). Nasal orbital fat is seen at tip of pointer

Forehead Myotomy (Muscle Stripping)

1. Identify the mimetic musculatures in the plane superficial to, the subperiosteal dissection, which can be directly accessed (Fig. 2.45). (These muscles were exposed in section "Subcutaneous Dissection" in another specimen.)
2. To do so, incise the periosteum, exposing the glabellar musculature. Extending the small incisions will assist in identification.

   They include the following (Fig. 2.9):

   (a) Procerus: The procerus muscle (Fig. 2.46) is a vertically oriented muscle in the glabellar region. The muscle originates from the fascia of the inferior portion of the nasal bones and inserts into the dermis between the eyebrows, between the paired frontalis muscles (Figs. 2.47 and 2.48).

> **Clinical Correlation**
> Contraction results in horizontal glabellar rhytids.

   (b) Corrugator Supercilii Muscle This muscle has two heads, a transverse and oblique head (Fig. 2.49). The transverse head originates from the medial aspect of the superior orbital rim (Fig. 2.50), and the oblique head originates from the superior portion of the medial orbital rim (Fig. 2.49). Each head inserts into the dermis just superior to the medial third of the brow and the beneath medial brow respectively.

> **Clinical Correlation**
> Contraction pulls the eyebrow medially and inferiorly, causing vertical and oblique rhytids in the glabellar region.

   (c) Depressor Supercilii muscle: The depressor supercilii muscle (Fig. 2.51) acts as a medial brow depressor. It originates along the frontal process of the maxilla above the medial canthal tendon and inserts into the dermis under the medial brow.

The muscles in the glabellar region are innervated by the frontal (temporal) branch or the zygomatic branches of the seventh cranial nerve.

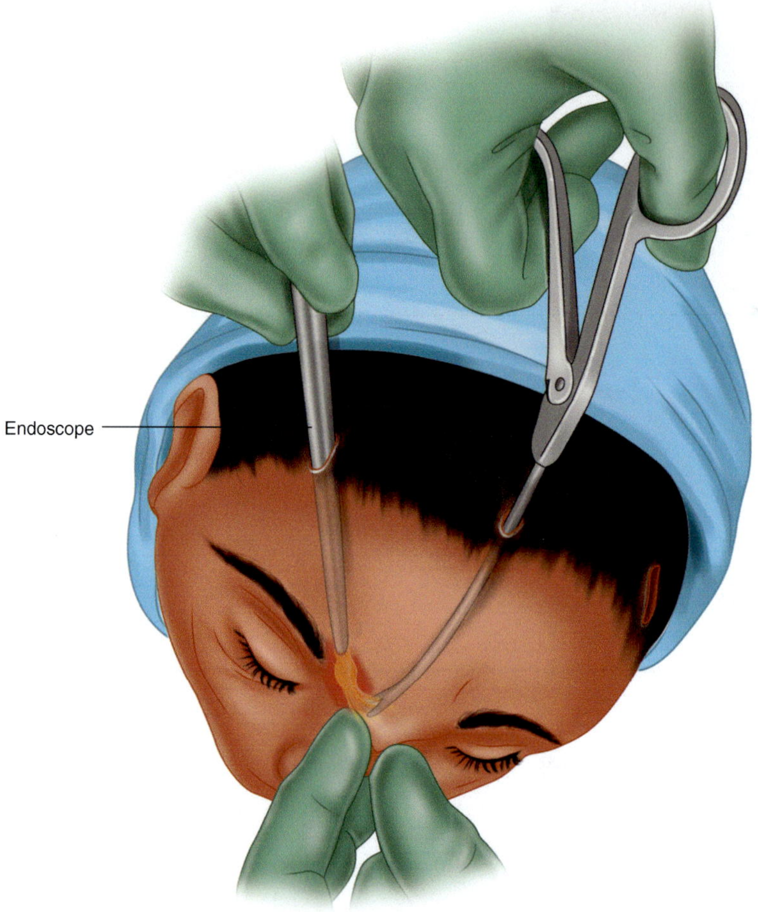

Fig. 2.45 Superior nasal orbital dissection and muscle release

3. Next release these muscles with curved forehead scissors. This is assisted using bimanual palpation during the dissection (Fig. 2.45).

Clinical and Anatomic Correlations
Clinically, this will weaken them and reduce their brow depressor function, thus allowing unopposed contraction of the intact frontalis muscles, to elevate the medial brow.

The facial musculature in the glabellar region have garnered attention as a frequent desired target of chemodenervation therapy.

Fixation for Brow Lift

After complete mobilization of the forehead and brow, two points of fixation for each brow are performed, one in the central zone and one in the temporal zone.

Clinical and Anatomic Correlation
For a youthful, natural unsurprised appearance, the peak or highest curve of the arch of each eyebrow should be at the level of the lateral canthus.

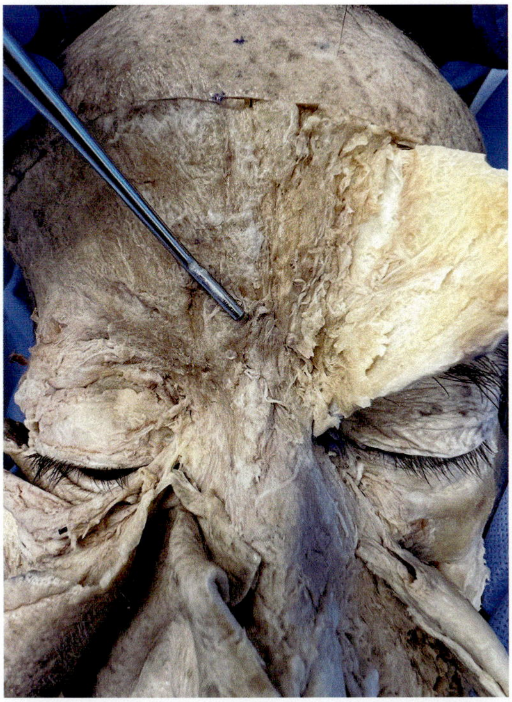

Fig. 2.46 The procerus muscle

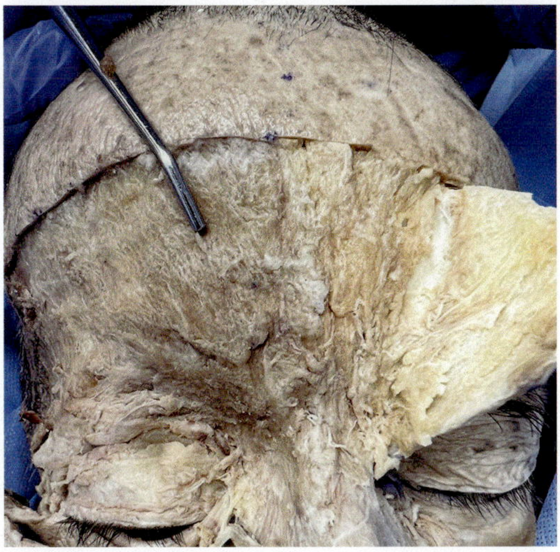

Fig. 2.47 Right frontalis muscle

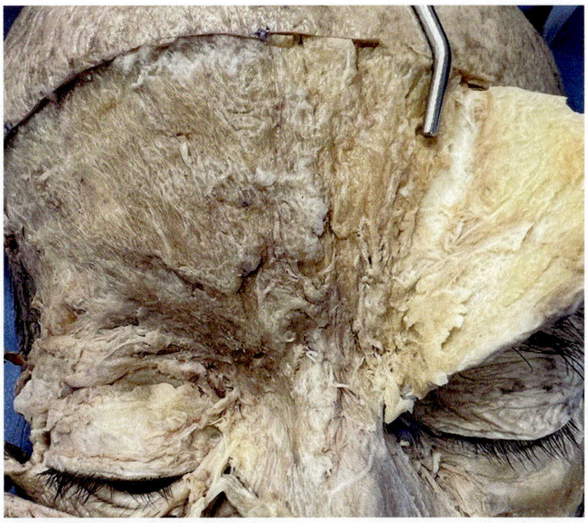

Fig. 2.48 Left frontalis muscle

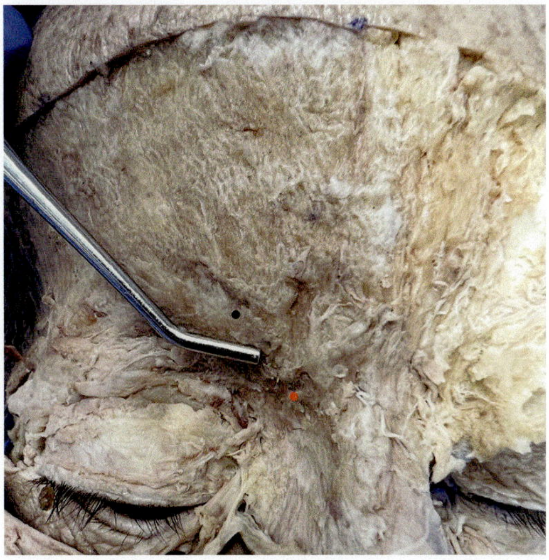

Fig. 2.49 Corrugator supercilii muscle. Transverse head (black dot) and oblique head (red dot)

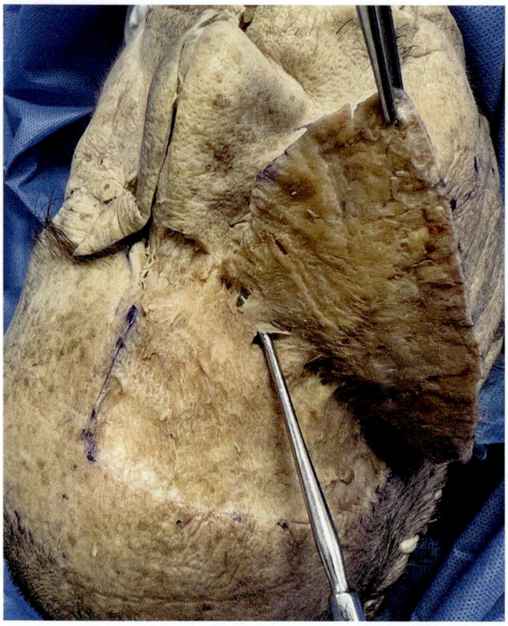

Fig. 2.50 Transverse head of corrugator supercilii muscle, on pointer, originating from medial aspect of the superior orbital rim

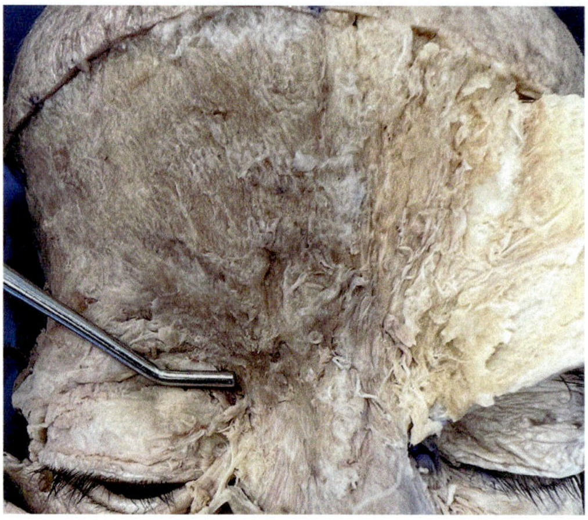

Fig. 2.51 Depressor supercilii muscle

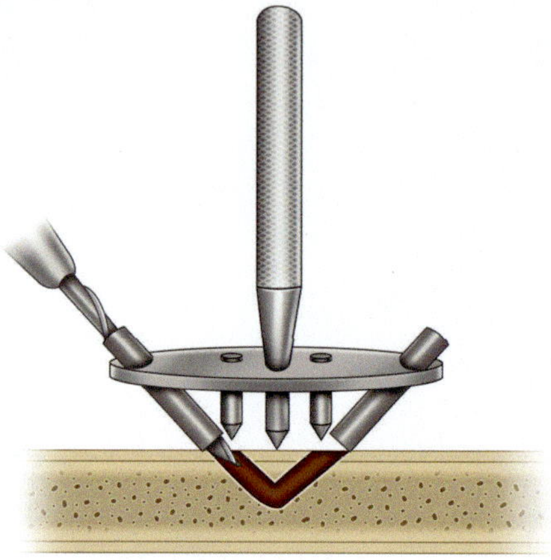

Fig. 2.52 Bone bridge

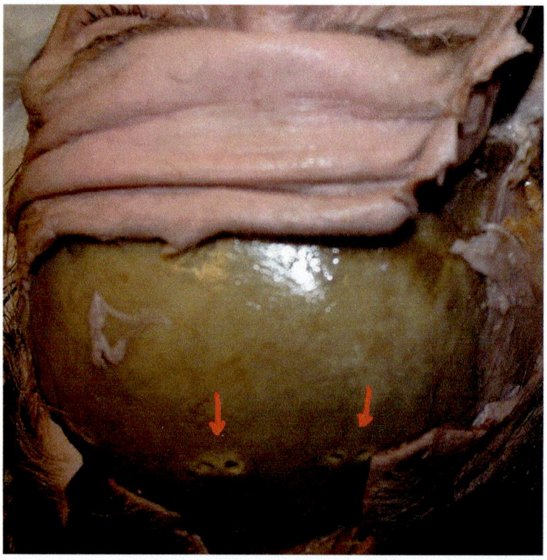

Fig. 2.53 Burr hole tunnels (red arrows) in bone of cadaver

Central Fixation

(a) For central fixation, through the paracentral scalp incision, use a brow lift bone bridge (Fig. 2.52) (Xomed) and drill to make a 4 mm depth bone tunnel in the diploic bone of the skull (Fig. 2.53). Alternatively, a specific drill can be used for placement of a resorbable fixation device (Endotine). Care is taken with fixation to ensure the thickness of the cranium is considered. At this location is it is about 8.1 mm thick.

(b) Pass a #2-0 polyethylene monofilament suture through the bone tunnel (Fig. 2.54).

(c) Pass the suture into the deep layers of the scalp (Fig. 2.55), then tighten to elevate the mobilized scalp.

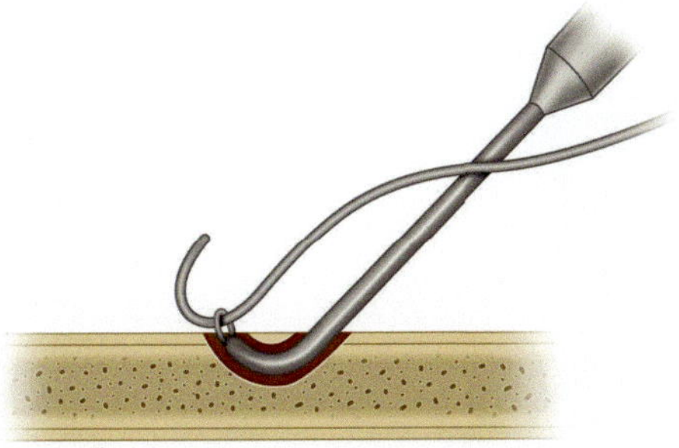

Fig. 2.54 Central fixation. Suture passed through bone tunnel

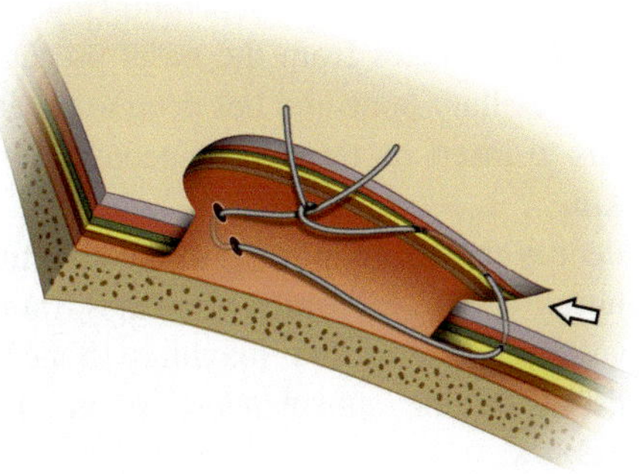

Fig. 2.55 Central fixation. Suture in burr holes and through deep layers of the scalp

(d) Close the incisions with surgical clips or sutures.

Temporal Fixation

(a) At the temporal incision, fixation is also performed. Use a 3-0 Vicryl suture or a #2-0 monofilament suture, in a mattress fashion, to fixate the superficial temporalis fascia inferiorly to the deep temporalis fascia superiorly (Fig. 2.56).

> **Clinical and Anatomic Correlation**
> When engaging the inferior aspect of the incision keep in mind the needle is passing through the superficial temporalis fascia. Care must be taken to avoid the frontal branch of the facial nerve, which is in the same plane.

(b) Secure the suture to the deep temporalis fascia with the desired degree of elevation.
(c) Close the incision in a layered fashion with deep 5-0 Monocryl, and superficial sutures or surgical clips.

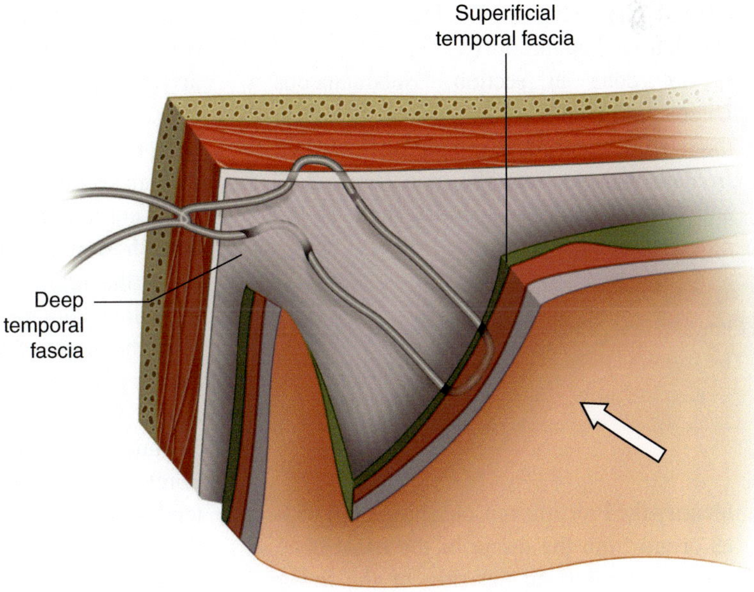

Fig. 2.56 Temporal fixation. The inferior edge of the incision with the superficial temporalis fascia is sutured to the deep temporalis fascia at the superior edge of the incision

Clinical Correlation
Facial nerve branches exit the parotid gland (see Chap. 3, Figs. 3.97 and 3.98). The frontal branch usually travels over the middle third of the zygomatic arch as 3–5 rami, and are in a deep, pre-periosteal plane. From here the nerve travels in a superior-medial direction, to a point 1.5 cm above the lateral end of the eyebrow (the Pitanguy line), transitioning from a deeper plane at the zygomatic arch to a superficial location, in the superficial temporalis fascia, above the arch.

The zygomatic branch of the facial nerve remains in a deep, submuscular plane after exiting the parotid, traveling beneath the zygomatico major muscle and going on to innervate the respective musculature of the face from the underside.

Convert the Dissection a to Bi-Coronal Approach

1. With a #10 or #15 blade, join the temporal and central incisions already oriented in the coronal plane (Fig. 2.57). Then reflect the skin-muscle flap inferiorly.
2. If not done in section "Subcutaneous Dissection" above, try to sharply dissect in the subcutaneous plane, separating the paired frontalis muscle from the skin (Figs. 2.47 and 2.48). Otherwise, identify them in the reflected forehead flap.

Clinical correlation
The frontalis muscle is the only muscle that elevates the brow.

3. Identify the Procerus muscle (Fig. 2.46) with its origin from the fascia of the nasal bone and its insertion on the skin of the lower forehead.

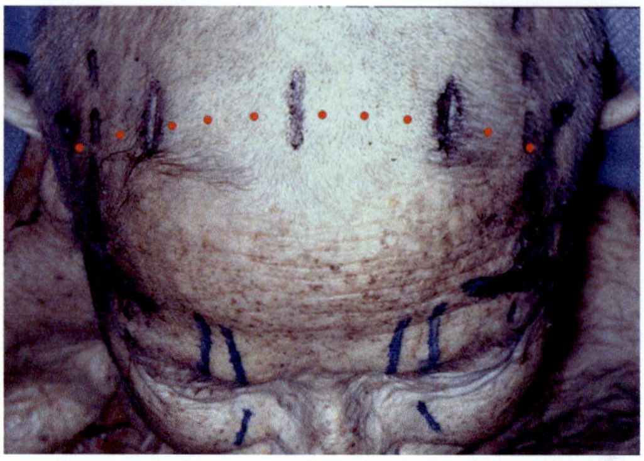

Fig. 2.57 Site of incision (red dots) for conversion to bi-coronal brow lift

4. Identify the corrugator supercilii (Fig. 2.49) which originates from the nasal process of the maxillary bone and lies deep to the frontalis to insert on the subcutaneous eyebrow skin.
5. Identify the orbital portion of the orbicularis muscle (Fig. 2.11) which originates from the nasal process of the maxillary bone and inserts on the subcutaneous tissue if the eyebrow.
6. Identify the depressor supercilii (Fig. 2.51) which are medial fibers of the orbicularis oculi muscle and insert on the subcutaneous eyebrow skin.
7. Next dissect the forehead flap in the subperiosteal plane anteriorly to the conjoint tendon at the temporal line of fusion (TLF) (Fig. 2.58). The conjoint tendon may have been totally or completely lysed endoscopically in section "Connection of the Temporal and Central Forehead Zones" above.
8. Note how it is a curved line on the skull along the origin of the temporalis muscle, extending from the supraorbital rim.
9. Note the origin of the deep temporalis fascia and its junction with the periosteum.
10. Next, if not already done in section "Connection of the Temporal and Central Forehead Zones", totally cut the conjoint tendon off the temporal line of fusion (Fig. 2.59).
11. Dissect to the supraorbital rim in the subperiosteal plane, with a Freer elevator. Identify

the supraorbital neurovascular bundle at the medial aspect of the supraorbital rim (Fig. 2.17).

12. Identify the arcus marginalis. Then incise it completely to the lateral canthus exposing the post septal orbital fat and the roof of the orbit.

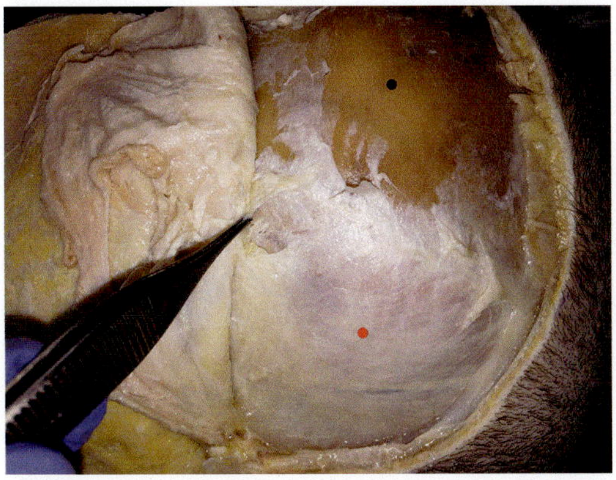

Fig. 2.58 Temporal line of fusion (TLF). Note the temporalis fascia and muscle (red dot), the frontal bone (black dot) and the lateral aspect of the supraorbital rim (pointer)

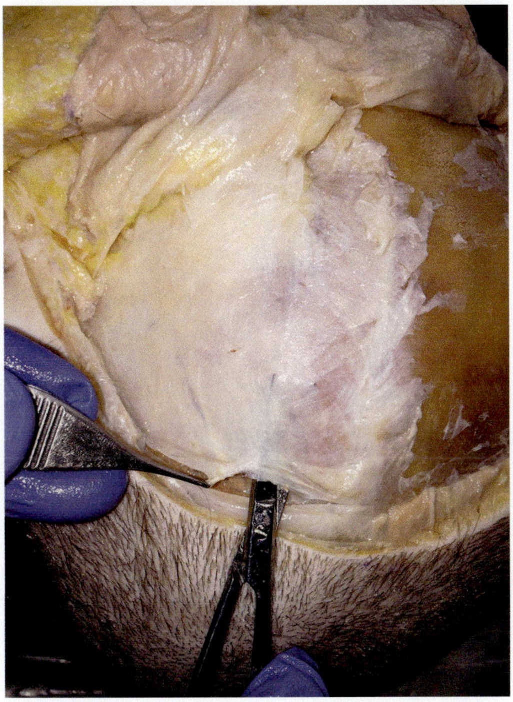

Fig. 2.59 Lysis of the conjoint tendon off the temporal line of fusion

Further Reading

Bedrossian EH, Della Rocca RC. Management of zygomaticomaxillary (tripod) fractures. In: Smith B, editor. Ophthalmic plastic and reconstructive surgery. St. Louis: Mosby Company; 1987. p. 512–5.

Bohr C, Bajaj J, Soriano RM, Shermetaro C. Anatomy, head and neck, temporoparietal fascia. Treasure Island, FL: StatPearls Publishing; 2022.

Cohn JE, Othman S, Bosco S, Shokri T, Evarts M, Papajohn P, Zwillenberg S. Management of isolated zygomatic arch fractures and a review of external fixation techniques. Craniomaxillofac Trauma Reconstr. 2020;13(1):38–44.

Jordan DR, Mawn L, Anderson RL. Forehead, eyebrows, eyelids, and canthi. In: Jordan DR, Mawn L, Anderson RL, editors. Surgical anatomy of the ocular adnexa: a clinical approach. 2nd ed. New York, NY: Oxford University Press; 2012.

Karimi N, Kashkouli MB, Sianati H, Khademi B. Techniques of eyebrow lifting: a narrative review. J Ophthalmic Vis Res. 2020;15(2):218–35.

Knize DM. Nerves and vessels of the forehead and temporal fossa. In: Knize DM, Drisko M, editors. The forehead and temporal fossa. Philadelphia, PA: Lippincott, Williams & Wilkins; 2001a.

Knize DM. Muscles of the forehead and temporal fossa. In: Knize DM, Drisko M, editors. The forehead and temporal fossa. Philadelphia, PA: Lippincott, Williams & Wilkins; 2001b.

Patrinely JR, Cech DA. Hemicoronal flap approach for lateral orbitotomy. Arch Ophthalmol. 1989;107(10):1421–2. https://doi.org/10.1001/archopht.1989.01070020495012.

Sykes JM. Endoscopic brow and surgical technique. Xomed; 1998. p. 1–10.

The Face

3

Edward H. Bedrossian Jr., Richard R. Schmidt, Bradley N. Lemke, Alison H. Watson, and Kareen Shebaclo

In this chapter, the dissection of the midface and lower face will proceed anatomically in a layered fashion starting with (1) surface anatomy and landmarks, (2) skin and subcutaneous fat, (3) subcutaneous fat (4) the superficial musculoaponeurotic system (SMAS) and muscles of facial expression, (5) sub-SMAS fat and retaining ligaments, (6) deep facial muscles of mastication, the facial nerve and parotid gland, and finally (7) the deep fat pads of the face. Clinical correlation is included.

A strong understanding of this anatomy will provide the reconstructive and aesthetic surgeon knowledge necessary to perform the most appropriate surgical technique for facial reconstruction and rejuvenation without threatening the form and function of the critical structures in the midface and lower face.

The *midface* is defined superiorly by a horizontal line extending from the lateral canthus to the medial canthus. Inferiorly, it is bordered by a line extending from the inferior edge of the tragus to the lateral aspect of the oral commissure (Fig. 3.1). The midface can be subdivided into anterior and lateral components by a line drawn from the lateral orbital rim to the oral commissure. The *anterior midface* refers to the "triangular" area between the lower eyelid and nasolabial fold. The *lateral midface* extends over the zygomatic arch and includes the zygomatic malar and submalar regions.

The *lower face* begins beneath the line extending from the tragus to the oral commissure. Its inferior extent is defined at the lower edge of the mandible, laterally from the ramus of the mandible to the midpoint of the chin.

Richard R. Schmidt has died before the publication of this book.

E. H. Bedrossian Jr., MD, FACS (✉)
Wills Eye Hospital, Sydney Kimmel Medical College of Thomas Jefferson University, Philadelphia, PA, USA

Department of Oculoplastic and Orbital Surgery, Wills Eye Hospital, Philadelphia, PA, USA

Clinical Professor Ophthalmology, Lewis Katz School of Medicine at Temple University, Philadelphia, PA, USA

R. R. Schmidt, PhD (Deceased)
Department of Pathology, Anatomy and Cell Biology, Sydney Kimmel Medical College of Thomas Jefferson University, Philadelphia, PA, USA

B. N. Lemke, MD, FACS
Lemke Facial Surgery, Madison, WI, USA

Department of Ophthalmology and Visual Sciences, School of Medicine and Public Health, University of Wisconsin-Madison, Madison, WI, USA
e-mail: lemke@lemkefacialsurgery.com

A. H. Watson, MD, FACS · K. Shebaclo, MD
Department of Oculoplastic and Orbital Surgery, Wills Eye Hospital, Philadelphia, PA, USA

E. H. Bedrossian Jr et al. (eds.), *Anatomy of the Forehead, Face, and Neck*,
https://doi.org/10.1007/978-3-031-56140-5_3

Fig. 3.1 Regions of the face

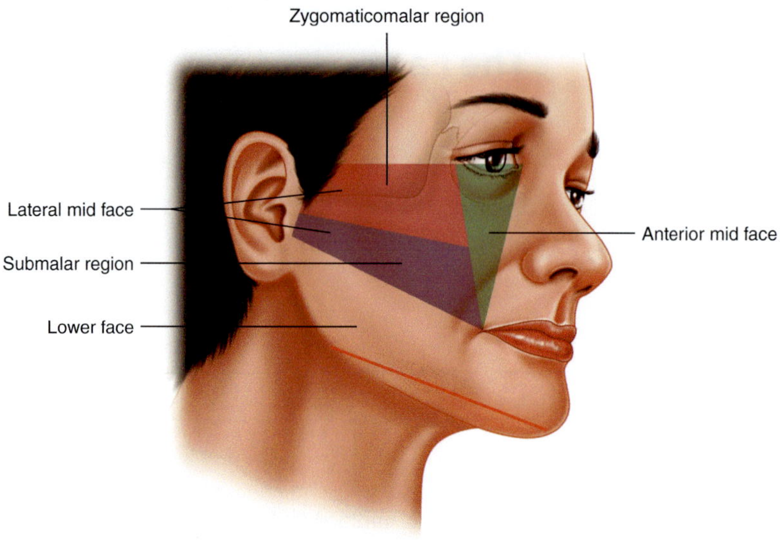

Fig. 3.2 Layers of the scalp and face. 1. Skin; 2. Subcutaneous tissue; 3. Frontalis muscle (forehead) or superficial musculoaponeurotic layer (face); 4. The loose areolar tissue (forehead) or retaining ligaments (face); 5. Periosteum (forehead) or deep fascia (face)

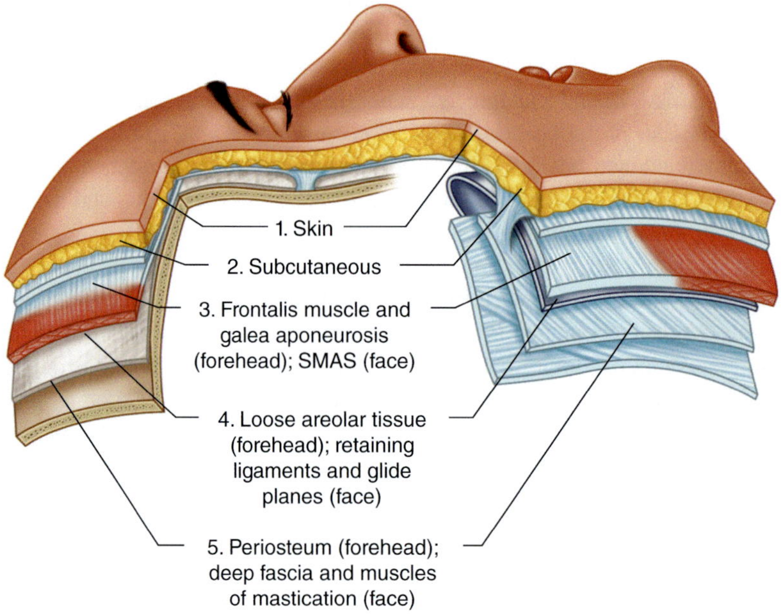

The soft tissue of the face is composed of five layers analogous to those present in the forehead and brow (Fig. 3.2) with the exception of the deep layer of the midface which is unique. While the periosteum is the deepest layer in the scalp, forehead and brow, the deepest layer in the midface is a fascial plane overlying soft tissue to include the parotid gland, the muscles of mastication, and the oral cavity.

Surface Anatomy and Landmarks

The midface displays three folds or creases (Fig. 3.3): the nasojugal fold, the malar fold, and the nasolabial fold. The lower face displays the mesolabial fold.

1. Identify the *nasojugal fold* (tear trough) located below the medial aspect of the inferior

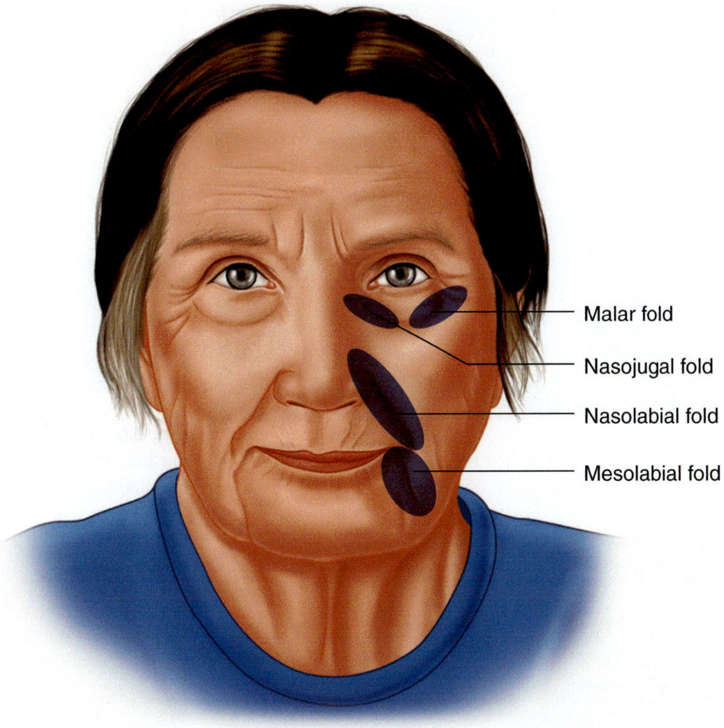

Fig. 3.3 Surface anatomy of the face

palpebral crease of the lower lid and extends inferolaterally at 45 degrees.

2. Identify the *malar fold* originating lateral to and below the lateral canthus at the junction of the maxilla and zygomatic bones. It extends inferomedially at 45° until it meets the nasojugal fold about 15 mm below the center of the lower lid margin.
3. Identify the *nasolabial fold* located below the medial aspect of the nasojugal fold, extending inferolaterally along the side of the nose toward the oral commissure.
4. Identify the *mesolabial fold* located below the oral commissure, extending inferiorlaterally over the mandible.

Clinical Correlation

In youth, the midface and lower face is full, and uniform, without evident folds or creases. However, with time, the contour of the midface and lower face deflates and descends, leading to the prominence of the aforementioned facial folds or creases.

Skin Incisions of Face, Nose, Mouth and Ear

The skin of the face is thin and firmly adherent to the underlying superficial fat and fascia in the midface, facilitating movement of the muscles and overlying skin as a single unit.

1. Mark the site of the skin incisions (Fig. 3.4).
2. With a no. 15 blade, a skin incision is made as marked, anterior to the tragus (Fig. 3.5), care taken not to disturb the underlying perichondrium in this thin skinned area.
3. Extend the incision inferiorly and wrap posteriorly around the ear lobe (Fig. 3.6).
4. Extend the incision starting medially from the tragus to the lateral canthus (Fig. 3.7), and then continue 2 mm below the eyelashes to the medial canthus.
5. At the medial canthus, extend the incision superiorly toward the gabella (Fig. 3.8) and continue in a "V pattern" above the height of

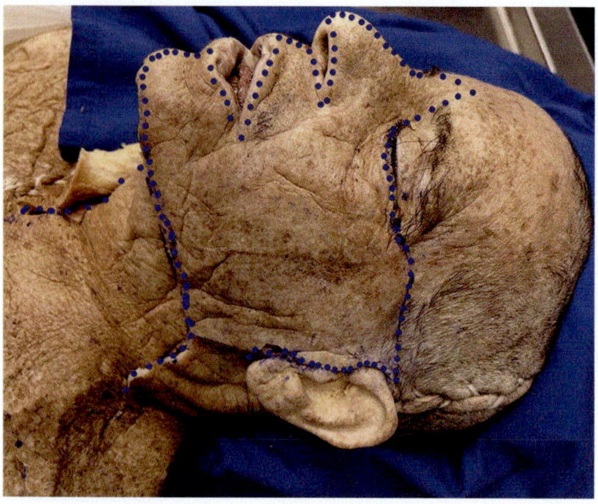

Fig. 3.4 Skin marking for incisions for face nose mouth and neck dissection

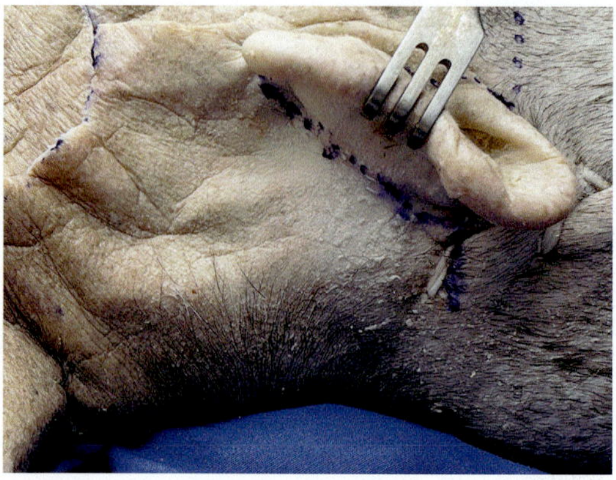

Fig. 3.6 Skin marking for retro-auricular incision. At the ear lobe the incision is extended post-auricularly over the conchal bowl toward the posterior hairline

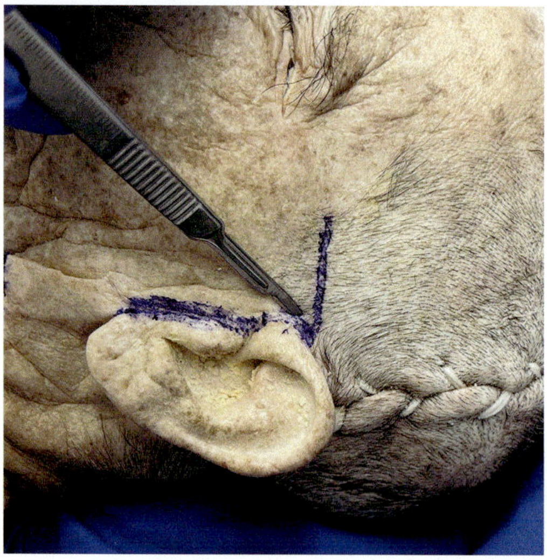

Fig. 3.5 Skin incision at the tragus. Skin incision beginning within the temporal hair tuft and extending inferiorly in the preauricular sulcus

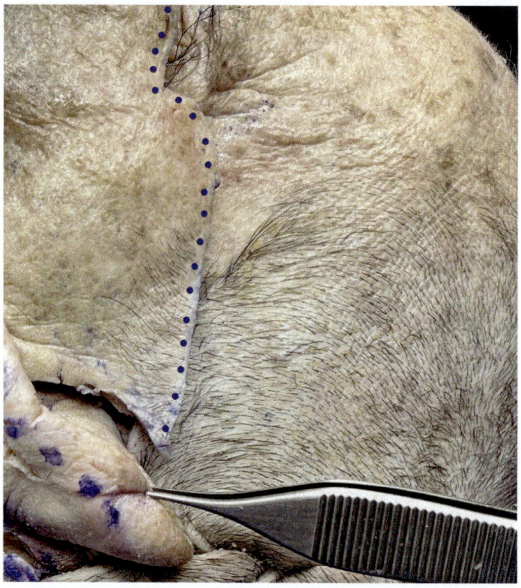

Fig. 3.7 Incision from the tragus medially to the lateral canthus, then below the lower eyelid margin

the brow (Fig. 3.9) fashioned similarly to the designed markings of a glabellar flap.

6. From the nasion, make a midline incision inferiorly along the bridge of the nose (Fig. 3.10) to a point superior to the upper lip (Fig. 3.11).
7. Carry the incision to encircle the mouth at the margin of the superior and inferior lips.
8. Make a midline incision from the inferior border of the lower lip to the mental protuberance of the chin.
9. Make an incision from the angle of the mandible extending along the inferior border of the mandible (Fig. 3.12) to the mental protu-

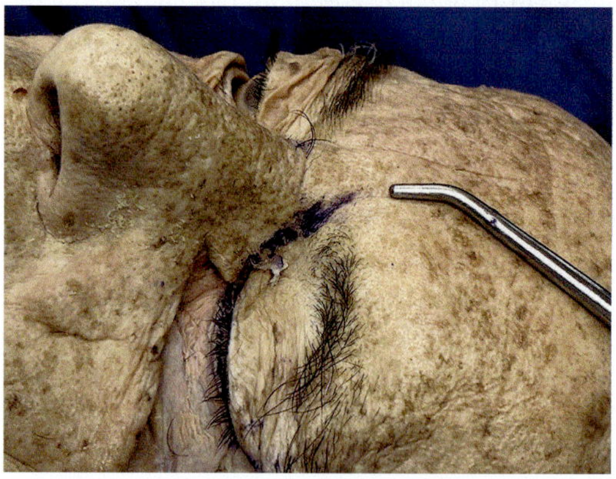

Fig. 3.8 Incision superiorly toward the gabella

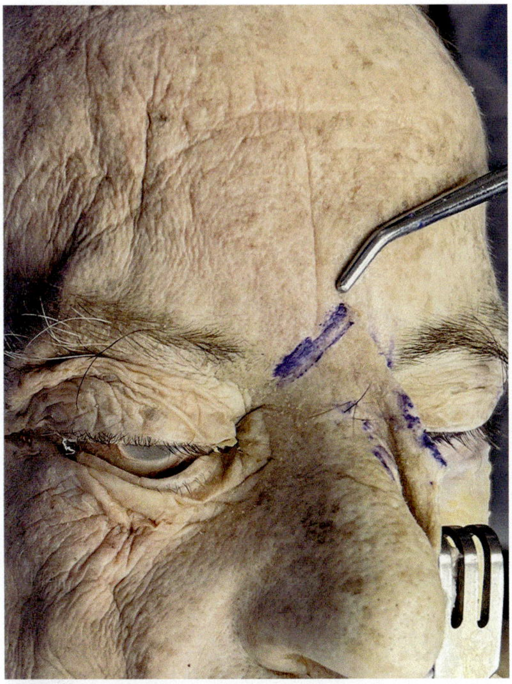

Fig. 3.9 "V pattern" above the brow

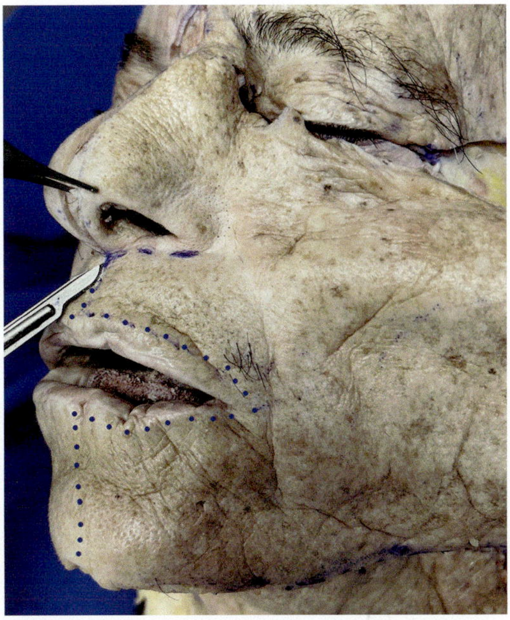

Fig. 3.11 Midline incisi`on from nasal tip to the upper lip

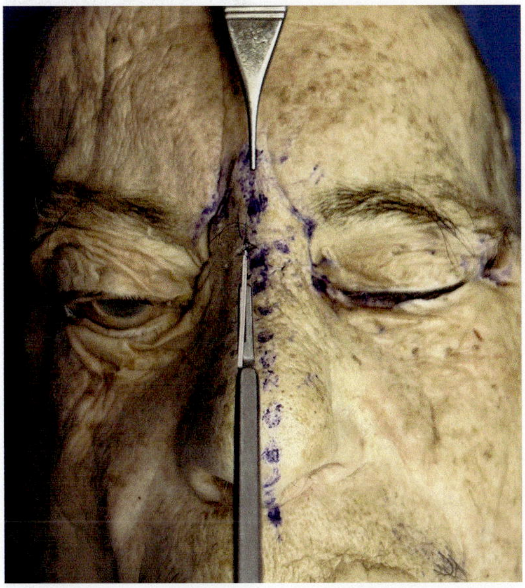

Fig. 3.10 Midline incision inferiorly along the bridge of the nose

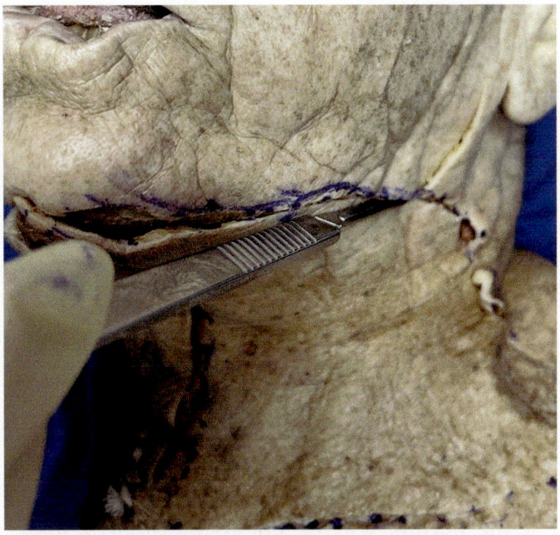

Fig. 3.12 Incision from the angle of the mandible extending along the inferior border of the mandible

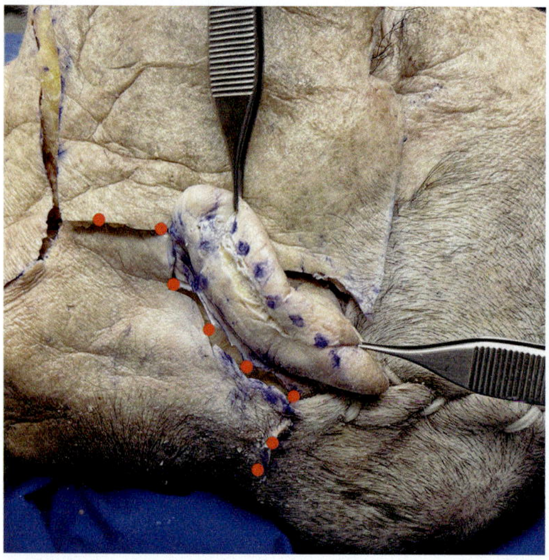

Fig. 3.13 Ear reflected showing retro-auricular incision (red dots)

berance of the chin. Note that this submental incision will be necessary for the neck dissection (Chap. 4).

10. Continue the incision in a retro-auricular fashion (Fig. 3.13) to enhance mobilization.

Subcutaneous Dissection

Midface

1. In the subcutanteous plane, starting laterally over the zygoma (Fig. 3.14), sharply dissect initially to raise the skin flap, then transition to blunt scissor dissection to a point 4 or 5 cm toward the cheek anteriorly (Fig. 3.15). Retinacular cutis attachments from the underlying fat and fibromuscular sheath to the dermis will be cut to facilitate release. Ensure care is taken to avoid going deeper into the underlying subcutaneous fatty layer and fibromuscular sheath.
2. If the skin of the lower eyelid has not been previously reflected, it must be done now, by carefully dissecting in the subcutaneous plane toward to the eyelid margin (Fig. 3.16). Note how the skin dramatically thins as the eyelid margin is approached. The eyelid skin is some of the thinnest in the body approximately 400 microns. For a detailed dissection of the eyelid,

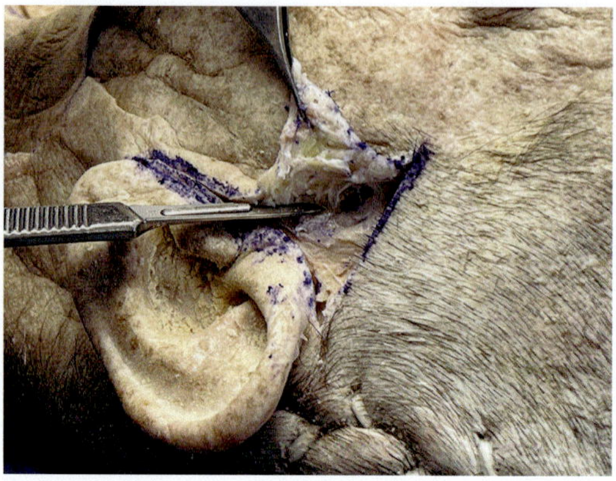

Fig. 3.14 Sharp subcutaneous dissection, starting laterally over the zygoma, note the reticular cutis attachments that need to be cut

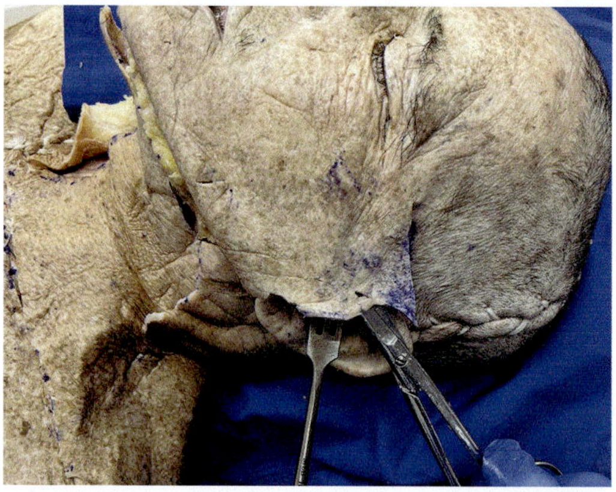

Fig. 3.15 Blunt subcutaneous dissection with spreading scissors continued 4 or 5 cm anteriorly

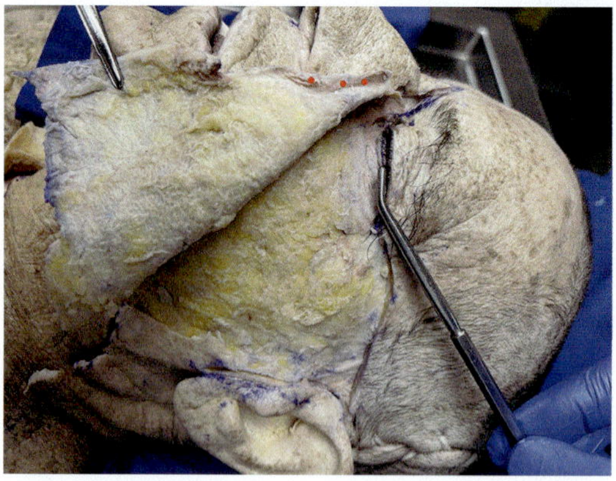

Fig. 3.16 Dissection in the subcutaneous plane of the cheek and eyelid to the eyelid margin. Note the thin reflected eyelid skin (red dots)

see manual one, Chap. 2 of this set "Surgical Anatomy of the Eyelids, Orbit and Lacrimal System: a dissection manual., Springer, 2022."

3. For better exposure, continue the subcutaneous dissection medially over the infraorbital rim toward the nasojugal fold (Fig. 3.17). Keep the cutaneous flap "on stretch" to assist with the sharp and blunt spreading dissection of the scissors.
4. Note the subcutaneous attachments at the nasojugal fold that need to be cut (Fig. 3.18).
5. Continue the subcutaneous dissection superiorly over the base of the nose (Fig. 3.19).
6. Identify the underlying muscles of the glabellar region to include the procerus muscle (Fig. 3.20). The glabella and nose will be studied further in the dissection below.
7. Continue the subcutaneous dissection inferiorly to over the body of the mandible (Fig. 3.21) toward the neck.
8. For improved exposure, with a 15 blade, extend the midline incision from the center of the chin, over the midline of the neck to the jugular notch of the sternum (Fig. 3.22).
9. Bluntly dissect and identify the superior portion of the platysma muscle along the entire inferior border of the mandible (Fig. 3.23).
10. Recall that the platysma muscle is a sheet of muscle covering the anterior neck. Continued subcutaneous dissection inferiorly and laterally will expose the platysma muscle in preparation for study of the neck in Chap. 4.

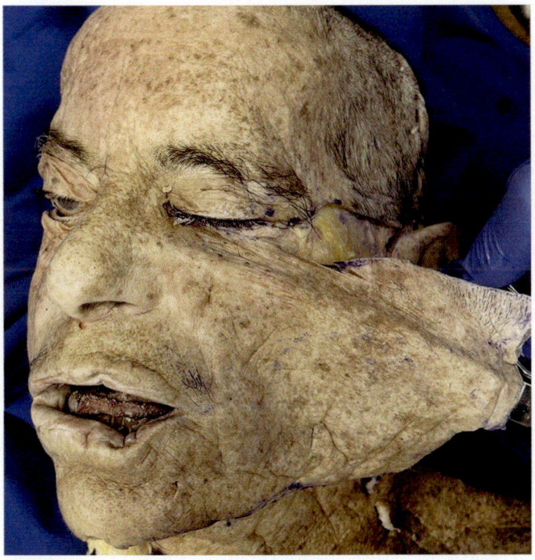

Fig. 3.17 Subcutaneous dissection medially toward the nasojugal fold

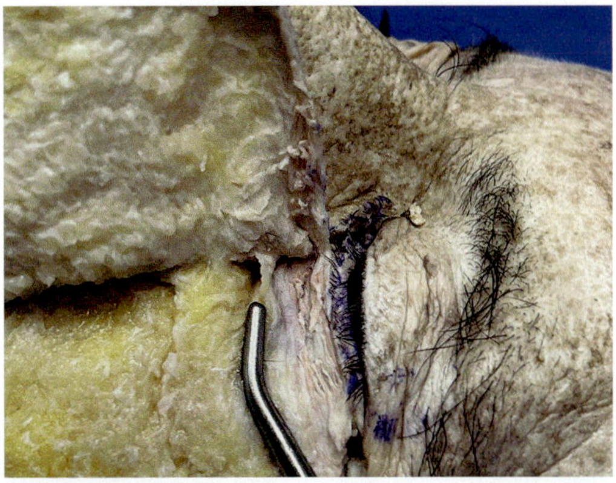

Fig. 3.18 Subcutaneous attachments at the nasojugal fold

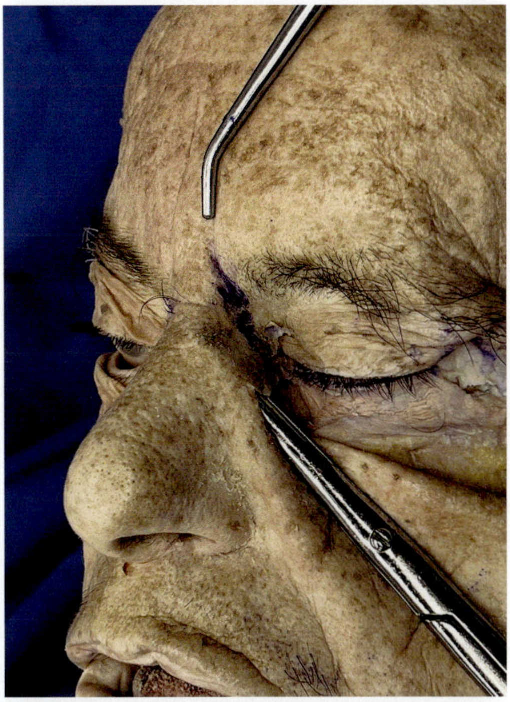

Fig. 3.19 Subcutaneous dissection superiorly over the base of the nose into the glabellar region

Nose

For easier cadaver dissection of retracted soft tissue of the nose a traction string can be placed if necessary, through the nares and reflected inferiorly.

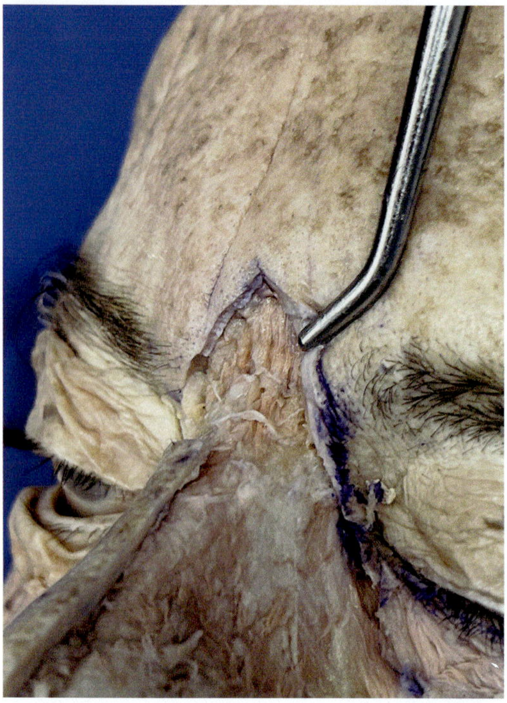

Fig. 3.20 Vertical fibers of the procerus muscle are demonstrated at the probe

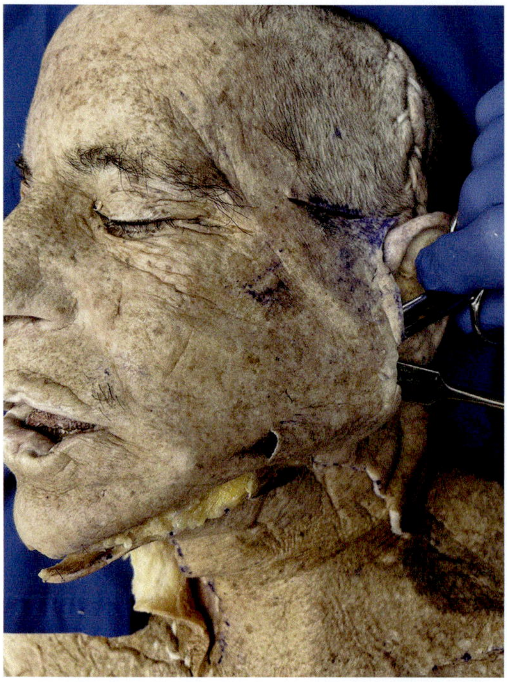

Fig. 3.21 Subcutaneous dissection inferiorly to over the body of the mandible

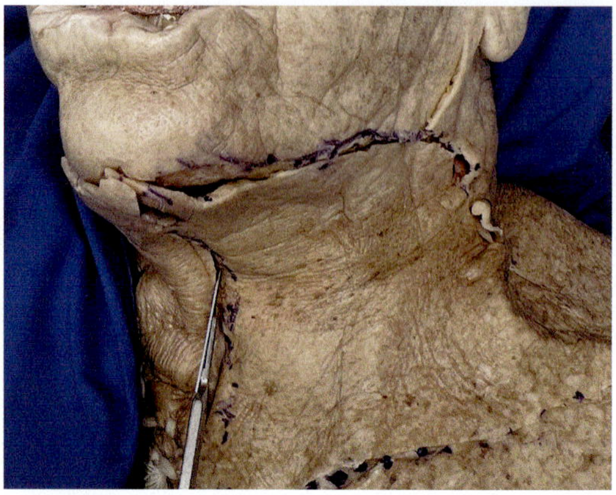

Fig. 3.22 Midline incision from the center of the chin, over the midline of the neck to the jugular notch of the sternum

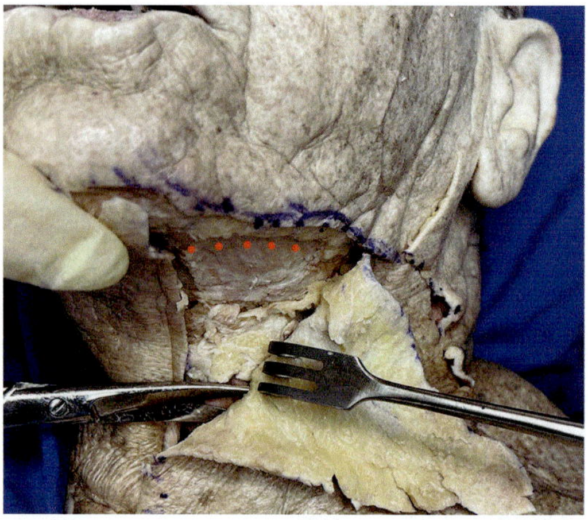

Fig. 3.23 Subcutaneous dissection onto the submandibular region and neck, exposing the platysma muscle (red dots) in the submandibular region

Muscles of the Nose

The group of nasal muscles of facial expression include the procerus (Fig. 3.20), the nasalis, the levator labii superioris alaeque nasi, and the depressor septi nasi muscles (Fig. 3.24)

1. Next, with lateral traction on the skin flap, and long dissection scissors, extend the subcutaneous dissection toward the frontal process of the maxilla onto the nasal bone (Fig. 3.25) and cartilages of the nose.
2. Expose the underlying *nasalis* muscle (Fig. 3.26). It is a paired muscle that covers

Fig. 3.24 Drawing of the muscles of the nose

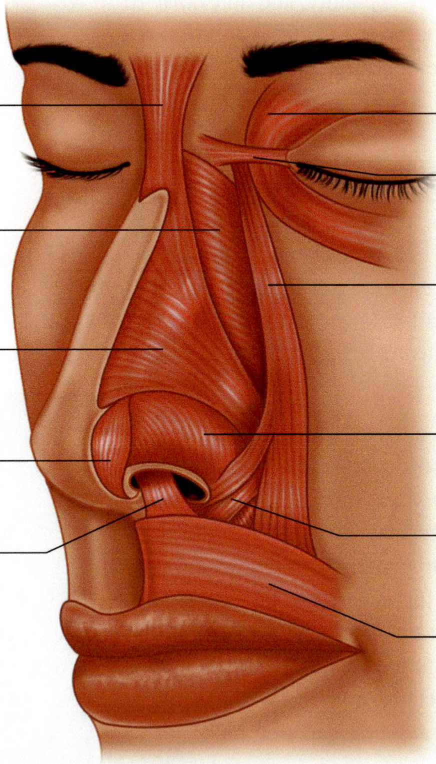

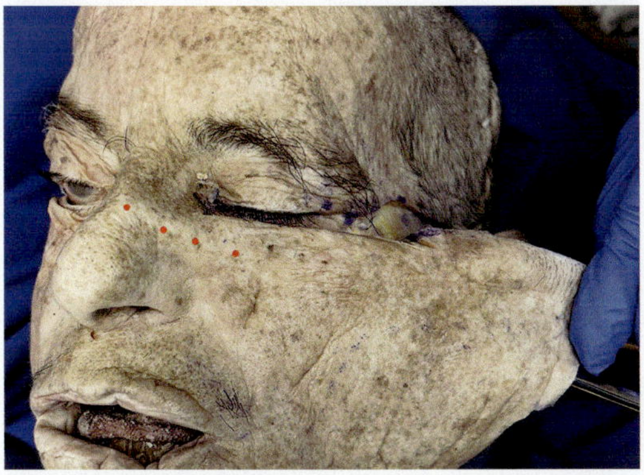

Fig. 3.25 Subcutaneous dissection onto the frontal process of the maxilla and nasal bone (red dots)

the dorsum of the nose. The nasalis muscle is innervated by the buccal branch of facial nerve (CN VII).

3. The nasalis muscle consists of two heads.

   First, identify *the transverse head* (also called the *compressor naris*), which originates on the maxilla, lateral to the incisive fossa and

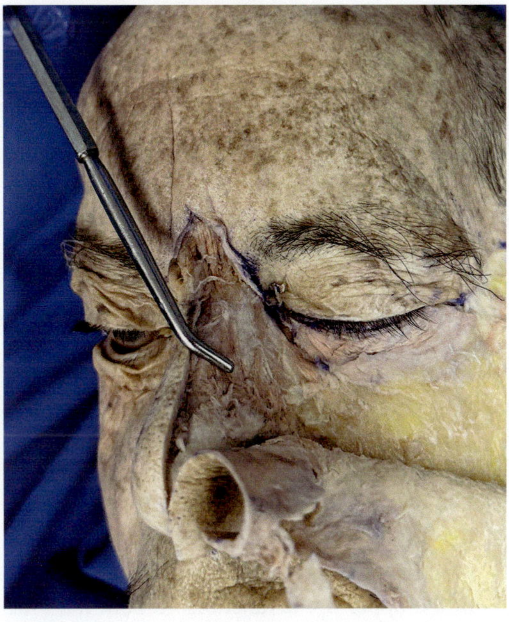

Fig. 3.26 Reflected subcutaneous skin flap exposes the underlying transverse head of the nasalis muscle (under probe)

extends superiorly, medially, and anteriorly to the bridge of the nose to join the transverse muscle from the opposite side.

Clinical Correlation
The transverse head of the nasalis compresses the nasal aperture, hence its other name compressor naris. In doing so, it wrinkles the nasal skin and is the site of Botox injections to treat the so-called Bunny Lines on the sides of the nose (Fig. 3.27).

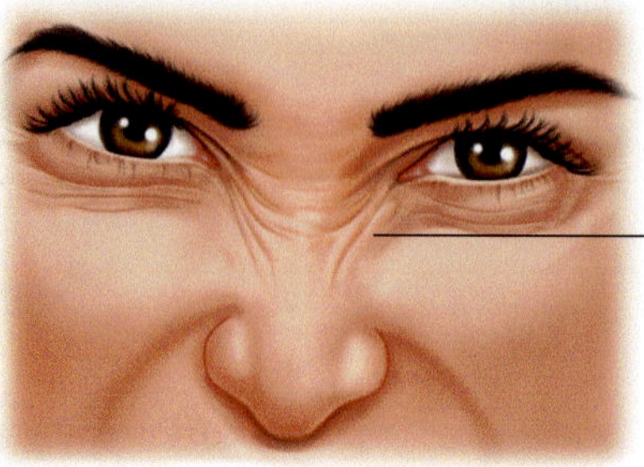

Fig. 3.27 "Bunny Lines" on the sides of the nose due to contraction of the transverse head of the nasalis muscle

Next, continue the subcutaneous dissection inferiorly to expose and identify the *alar head* (also called *dilator naris*) (Fig. 3.28). It attaches the greater alar cartilage to the skin at the point of the nose. It originates from the frontal process of maxilla, just superior to the lateral incisor. After a short superoanterior course, it inserts superior to the lateral crus of the major alar cartilage. Here, note how some fibers blend with the transverse part of nasalis.

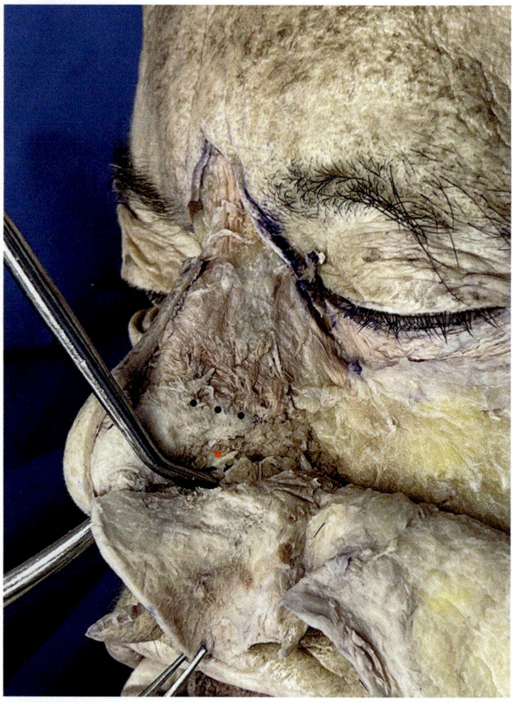

Fig. 3.28 The nasalis muscle. Note the alar head of the nasalis muscle (Alar nasalis) at the tip of pointer and red dot. It inserts superior to the lateral crus of the major alar cartilage under the pointer. Fibers blend (black dots) with the transverse head of nasalis, above

Clinical Correlation
The alar head of the nasalis muscle, moves the ala nasi cartilage (nostril wings) laterally and dilates the nostrils. These actions enable flaring of nostrils, which occurs during breathing and is emphasized in various emotionally driven situations. Nose bridges are occasional worn by athletes to assist in nasal dilation to enhance airflow into the nose.

4. Identify the *levator labii superioris alaeque nasi* (Fig. 3.29). It originates from the upper frontal process of the maxilla, courses inferiorly along the side of the nose. It then divides into a wider medial head which inserts onto the skin of the lateral nostril and a narrower longer lateral head which inserts onto the skin of the upper lip. It functions to both flare the nostril and elevate the lip.
5. Identify the small *depressor septi* nasi muscle (Fig. 3.30) which arises from the incisive fossa of the maxilla; its fibers ascend to insert onto the ala and septum of the nose and assist with constriction of the nares.

Clinical Correlation
The blood supply to the group of nasal muscles come from the superior labial, septal and lateral nasal branches of facial artery, and the infraorbital branch of maxillary artery (Fig. 3.31). These are a "danger zones" for injection of fillers to correct nasal bridge deformities or adjust lip contour in minimally invasive procedures.

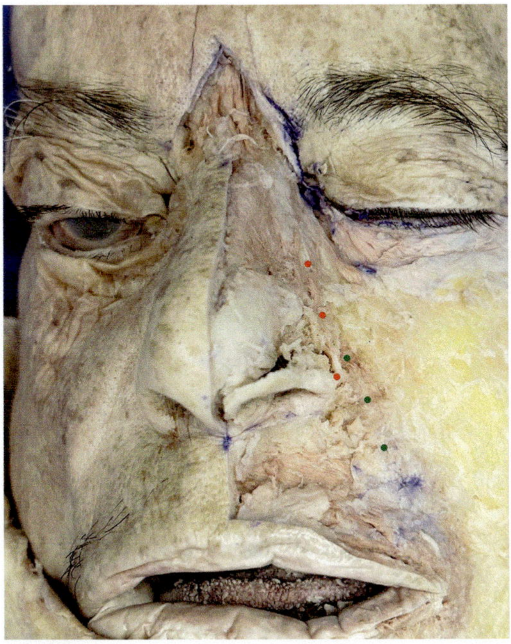

Fig. 3.29 The levator labii superioris alaeque nasi. Note the wider medial head (red dots) to the skin of the lateral nostril and a longer narrow lateral head to the upper lip (green dots)

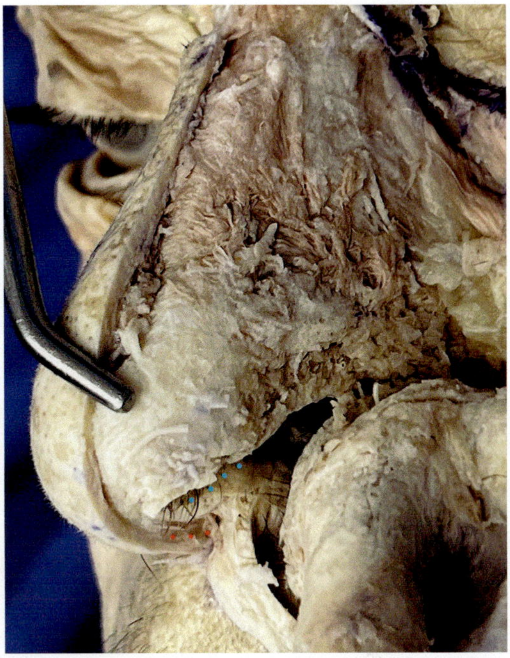

Fig. 3.30 Depressor septi nasi muscle (red dots). Note the alar cartilage at the pointer and the nasal septum (blue dots)

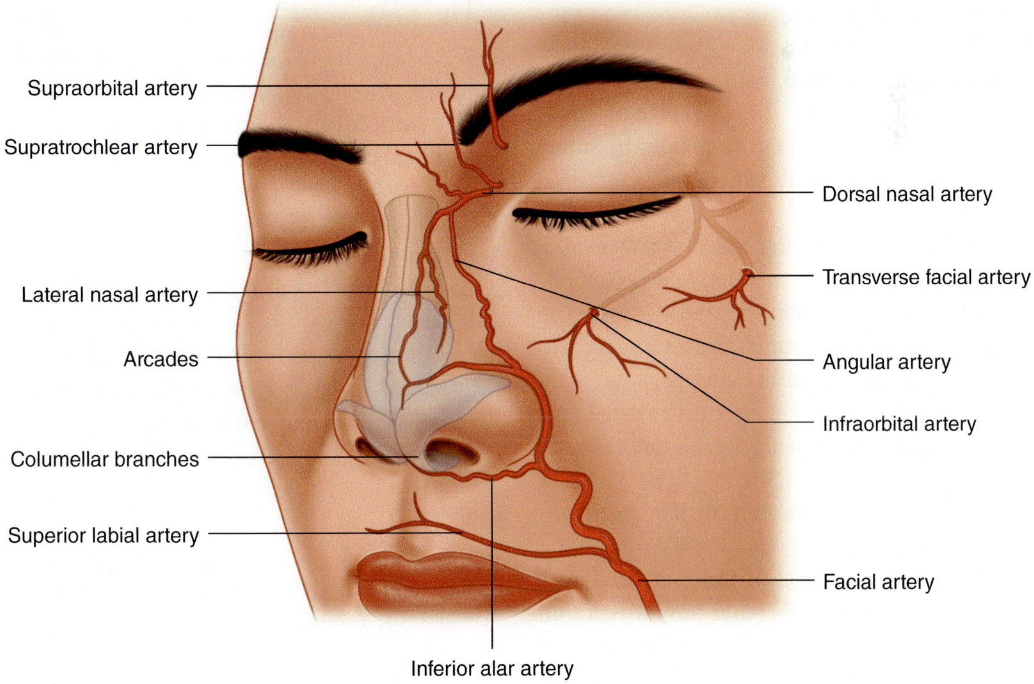

Fig. 3.31 The blood supply to the group of nasal muscles

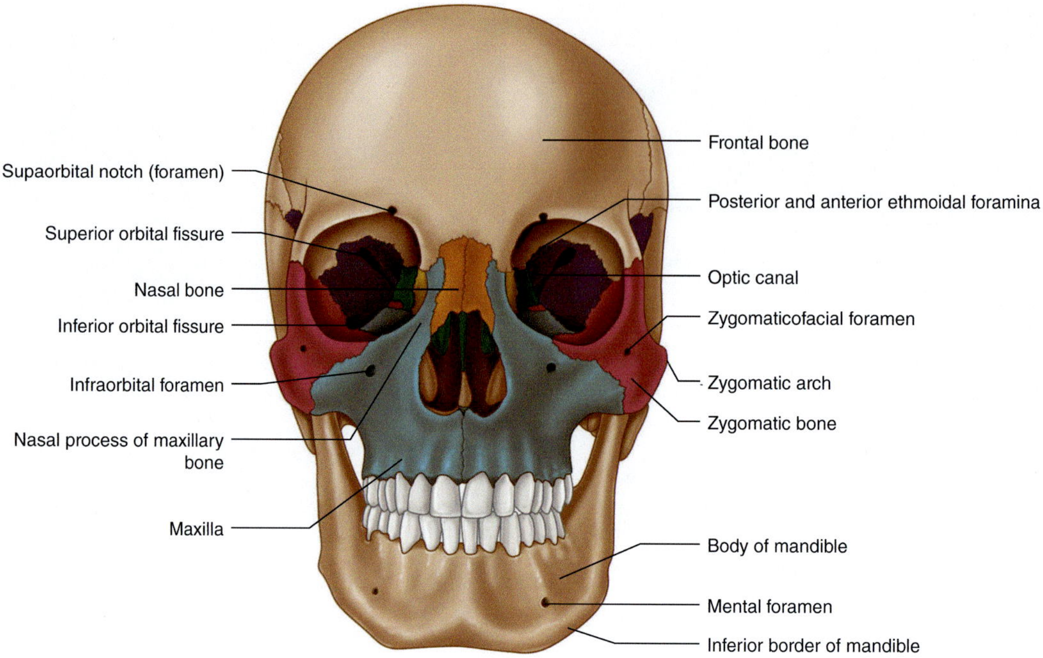

Fig. 3.32 Bones of nose and face

Bone and Cartilages of the Nose

1. Deep to the transverse head of the nasalis muscle, dissect to expose and identify the *nasal bone* (Fig. 3.32).
2. Continue the submuscular dissection inferiorly beyond the nasal bone, exposing the *lateral nasal cartilage* (Figs. 3.33 and 3.34). Note that it is fixed to the nasal bone by suture and continuous with the septal cartilage medially.
3. Continue the dissection inferiorly to expose the narrow *Sesamoid cartilages.* Inferior retraction at the nares may be necessary to better expose and separate the sesamoid cartilages from the alar nasal cartilage.
4. Continue the dissection inferiorly to the lower part if the nose, exposing the *Alar nasal cartilage* (Figs. 3.34 and 3.35).
5. Sharply separate the paired alar cartilages and retract laterally to identify its lateral crus and medial crus of the alar cartilages (Figs. 3.36 and 3.37). Note how it is a thin and flexible, mobile U-shaped plate bent in such a way to form both the medial and lateral wall of the nostril on its own side.
6. Further expose the midline Septal cartilage (*see* Fig. 3.36) extending from the lateral cartilage above, coursing medial to the sesamoid cartilage and alar cartilage ending with fibro-areolar tissue at the nasal tip (*see* Fig. 3.34).
7. Note how the nasal bone, and cartilages are paired with the opposite side.
8. The nasal cartilages are hyaline cartilage. The cartilage of the ear is elastic cartilage.

Clinical Correlation

Knowledge of nasal bone and cartilage anatomy is required by the cosmetic and functional rhinoplasty surgeon in the management of deformities of the nasal dorsum, nasal septum, and nasal tip.

Ear

1. Examine the external ear structures (Figs. 3.38 and 3.39) and identify the following:
   (a) Pinna
   (b) Helix
   (c) Antihelix
   (d) Lobule
   (e) Tragus

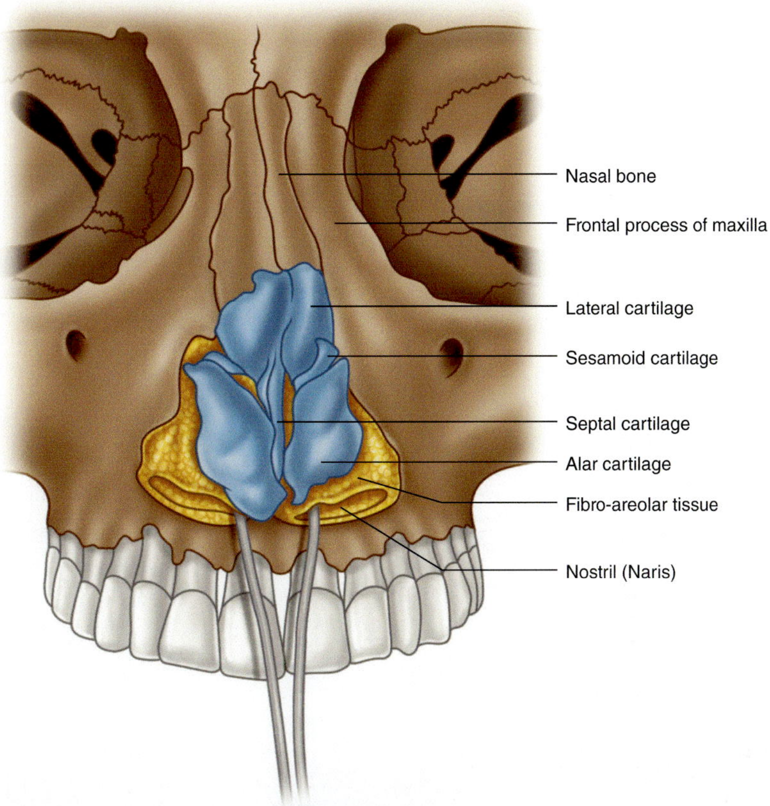

Fig. 3.33 Cartilages of the nose

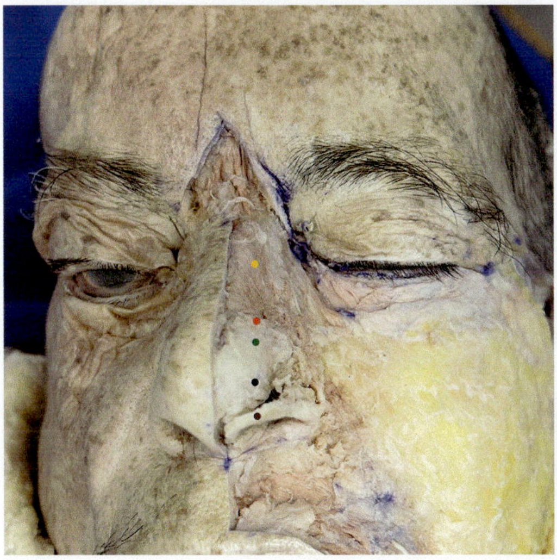

Fig. 3.34 Nasal cartilages. The nasal bone is not exposed but is deep to the nasalis muscle (yellow dot). Note the Lateral cartilage (red dot), the Sesamoid cartilage (green dot), the Alar cartilage (black dot), and the fibro-areolar tissue at the nasal tip (brown dot)

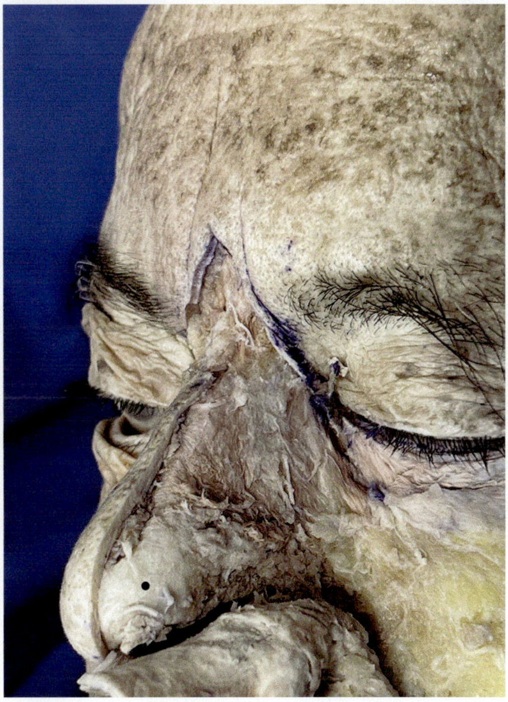

Fig. 3.35 Alar cartilage. Note the black dot on the lateral crus

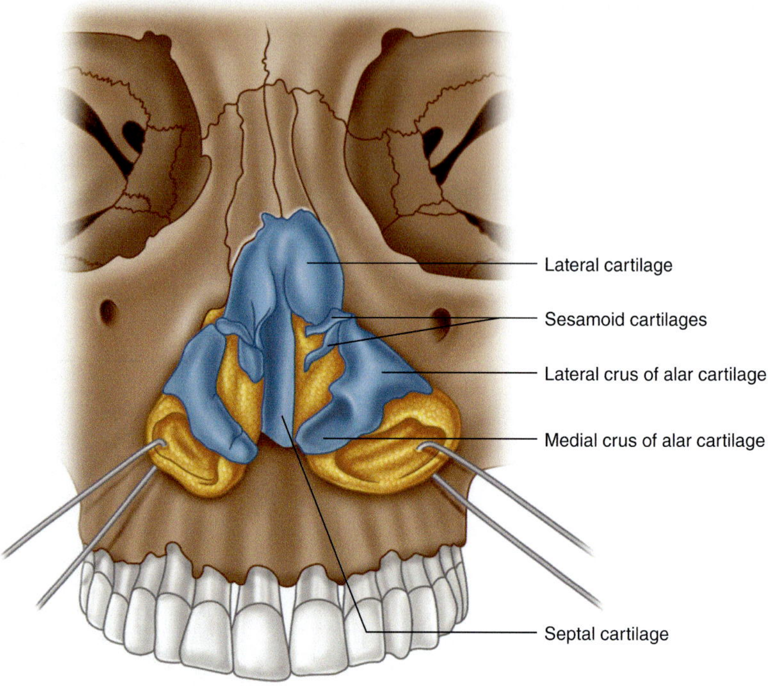

Fig. 3.36 Septal cartilage; lateral crus and medial crus of alar cartilage

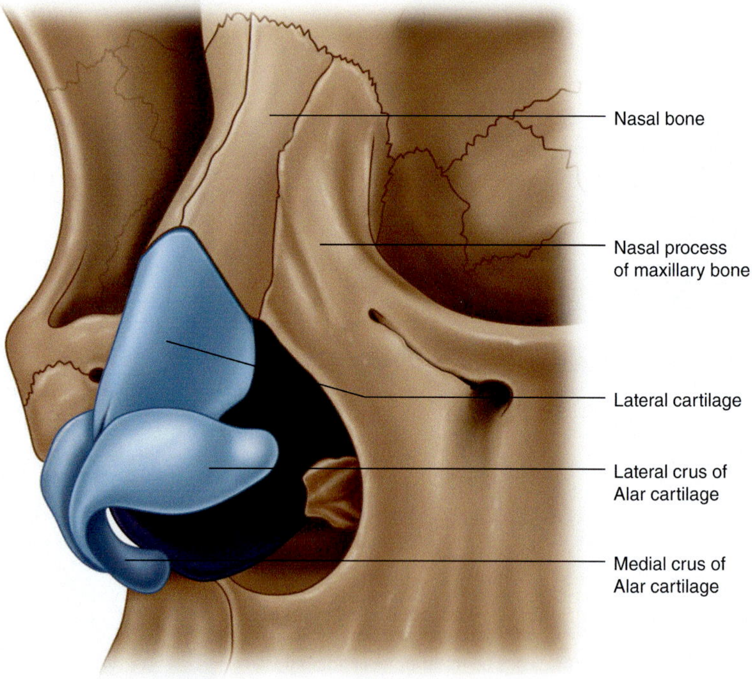

Fig. 3.37 Nasal bone, lateral cartilage, and alar cartilage

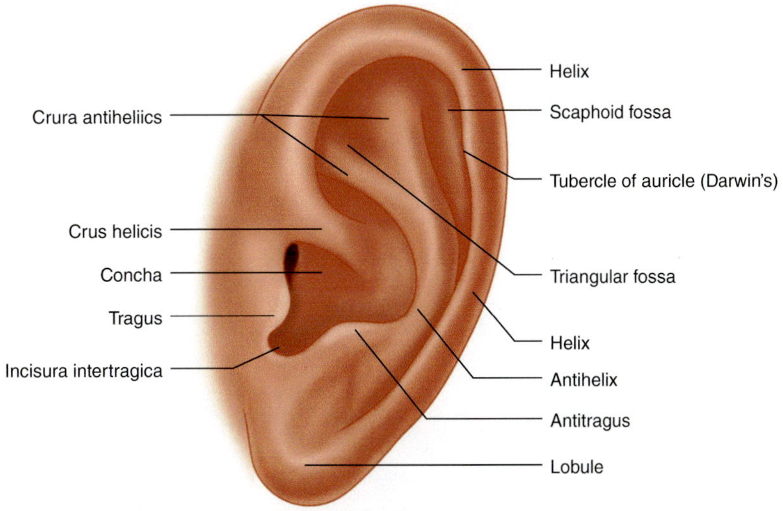

Fig. 3.38 External ear (pinna)

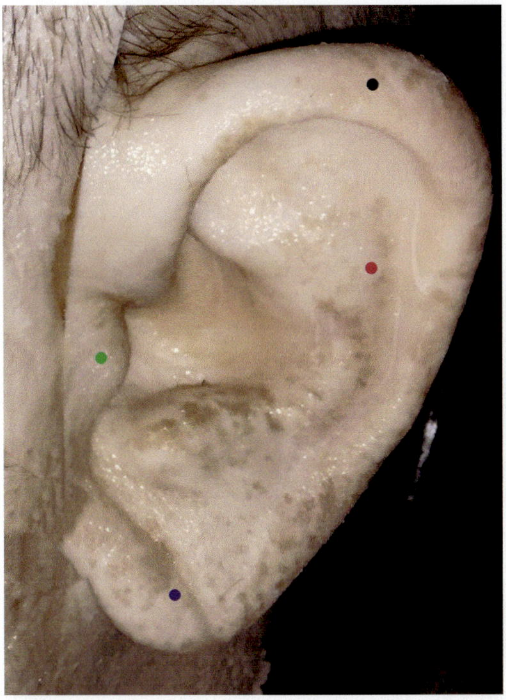

Fig. 3.39 The external surface anatomy of the ear is demonstrated. Note the helix (black dot), antihelix (red dot), tragus (green dot), and lobule (purple dot)

2. Note that there is no cartilage in the lobule.

Clinical Correlation
Torn earlobes are occasionally seen from pierced earrings.

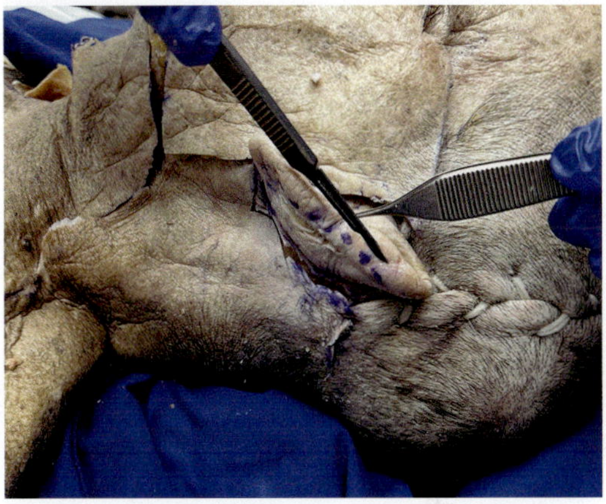

Fig. 3.40 #15 blade showing skin incision site at the helix

3. With a 15 blade, on the lateral surface of the helix (Fig. 3.40), make an incision through the skin exposing the yellowish elastic cartilage of the helix. Note that is very little subcutaneous tissue and the skin adheres to the cartilage (Fig. 3.41).

Clinical Correlation
It is this cartilage that can be harvested and used as an autograft for support in eyelid reconstruction and lid retraction surgery

4. Further dissect inferiorly in the subcutaneous plane to expose the stylomastoid area (Fig. 3.42).

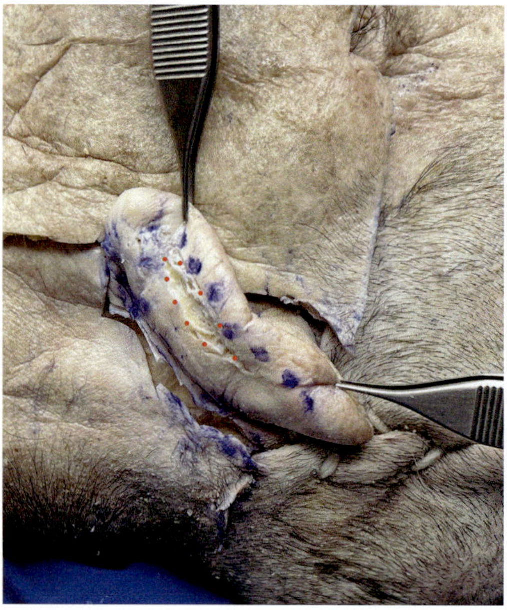

Fig. 3.41 Incision at helix through adherent skin and subcutaneous tissue (red dots) exposing elastic ear cartilage

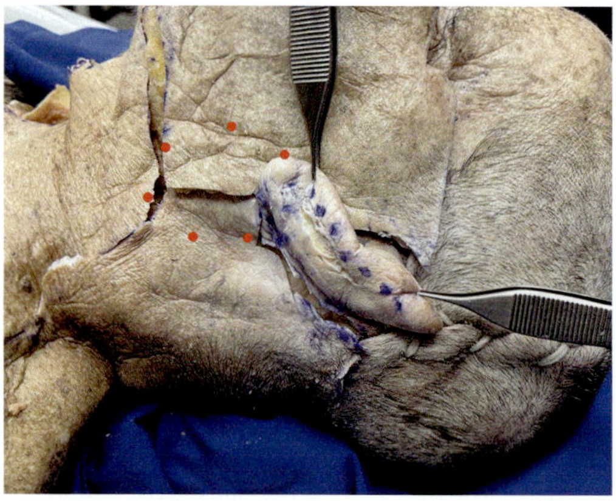

Fig. 3.42 Site of sub cutaneous dissection exposing the stylomastoid area (red dots)

5. Next retract or sew the helix of the ear forward to assist with exposure of the retro-auricular area.
6. In a subcutaneous fashion, elevate the retro-auricular skin (Fig. 3.43). Note how there is more subcutaneous tissue and is more mobile.

Clinical Correlation

The retro-auricular skin is an excellent source as a free skin graft for anterior lamella eyelid surgery.

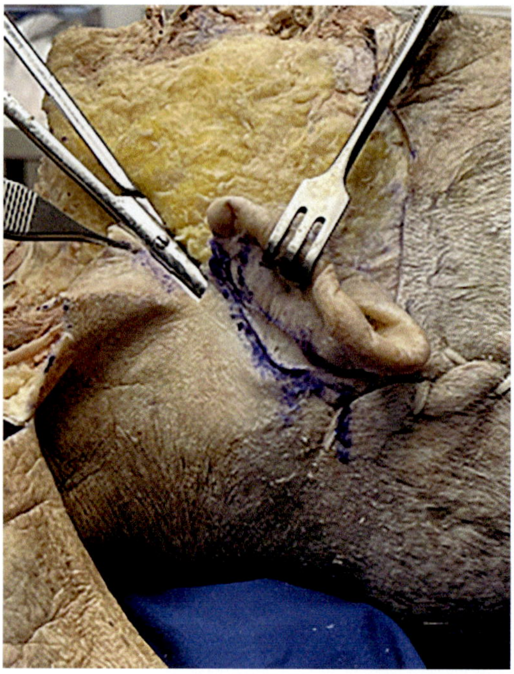

Fig. 3.43 Scissors in subcutaneous plane showing retro-auricular dissection along the previously incised retro auricular incision line

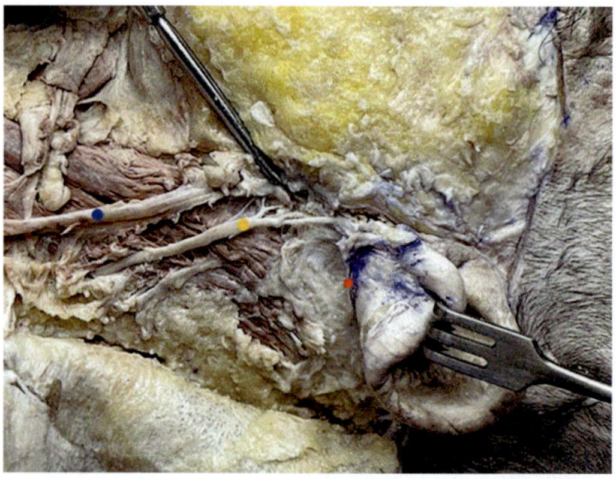

Fig. 3.44 The Great auricular nerve (yellow dot) ascending over the sternocleidomastoid muscle. Also note the external jugular vein (blue dot) and thin posterior auricular nerve (red dot)

7. Identify the posterior auricular nerve (Fig. 3.44), an extracranial branch of the facial nerve, arising near the stylomastoid foramen and runs upwards in front of the mastoid process.
8. With deeper dissection, identify the great auricular nerve, ascending along the sternocleidomastoid muscle (Fig. 3.44). It is derived

from the vagus nerve. It sends a branch to communicates with the posterior auricular nerve.

9. Identify the external jugular vein (Fig. 3.44).

Clinical Correlation

Knowledge of the retro-auricular and stylomastoid areas are important in performing facelift surgery as the greater auricular nerve is vulnerable to injury during this dissection.

Subcutaneous Fat Dissection

1. With the skin removed, but superficial to the muscles of facial expression identify the subcutaneous plane of fat (Fig. 3.45).
2. Note that it regionally varies in thickness. In the lower eyelid, no fat is present in the subcutaneous plane, while a moderate degree of fat is present in the midface (Fig. 3.46).
3. Identify the subcutaneous malar fat pad and its regions (Fig. 3.47). It is the subcutaneous fat layer of the midface. This continuous fat layer is somewhat arbitrarily divided into the following named compartments: nasolabial, medial, central, and lateral.

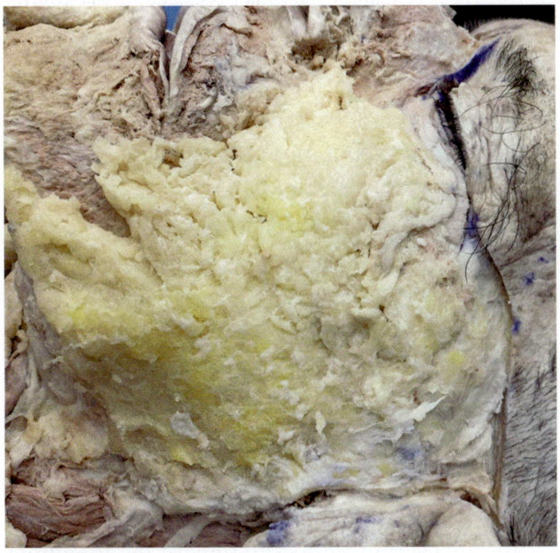

Fig. 3.45 Sheet of subcutaneous fat

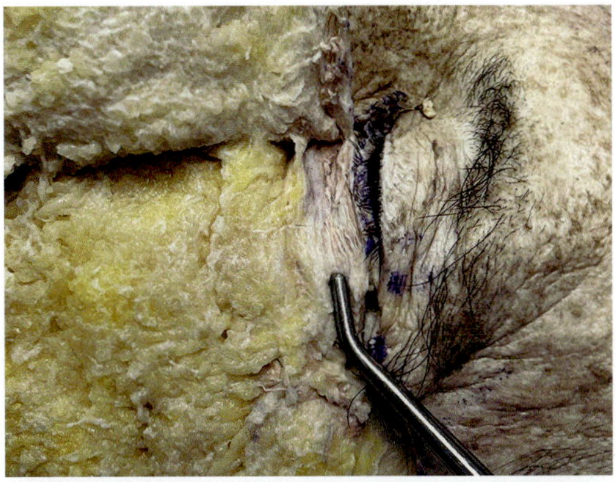

Fig. 3.46 Regional variation in thickness of subcutaneous fat. There is no subcutaneous fat at the preseptal and pretarsal lower lid, as the orbicularis is readily seen (pointer), while a moderate degree of fat is present in the midface

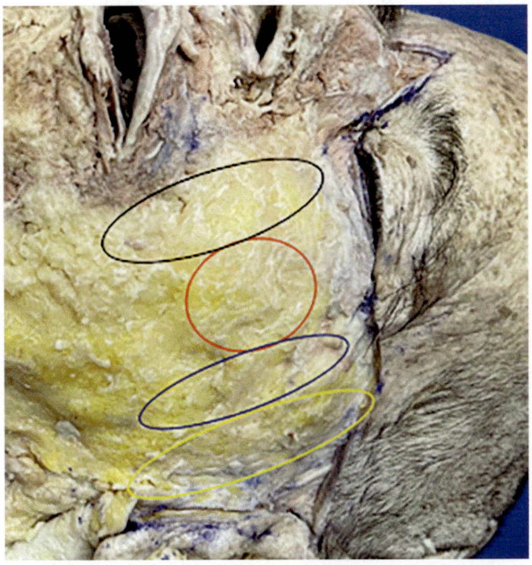

Fig. 3.47 Beneath the skin the superficial subcutaneous malar fat pad is seen with approximate locations of the named divisions of this continuous layer. Displayed are the nasolabial (black), the medial (red), the central (blue), and lateral (yellow) are shown

Clinical Correlation

The malar fat pad accounts for malar prominence in youth but descends with time. Interdigitation of the superficial fat with the underlying SMAS facilitates surgical mobilization of the skin, subcutaneous fat, and superficial fascial layers as a single aesthetic unit.

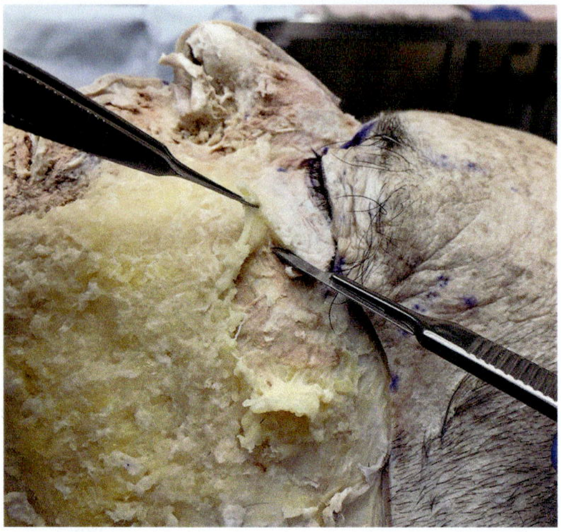

Fig. 3.48 Sharp dissection of composite fat and SMAS at infraorbital rim

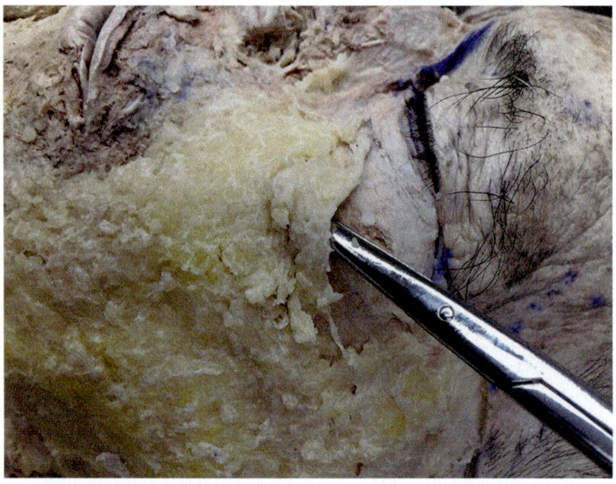

Fig. 3.49 Blunt dissection of composite fat and SMAS with spreading scissors under superior medial portion of subcutaneous malar fat pad

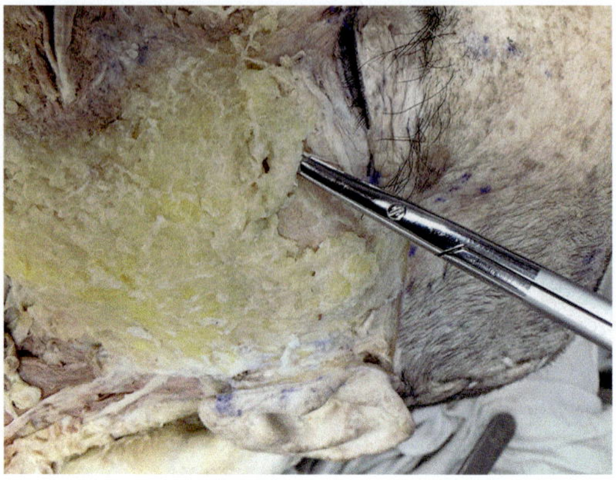

Fig. 3.50 Sub-composite fat and SMAS dissection inferiorly toward the oral commissure

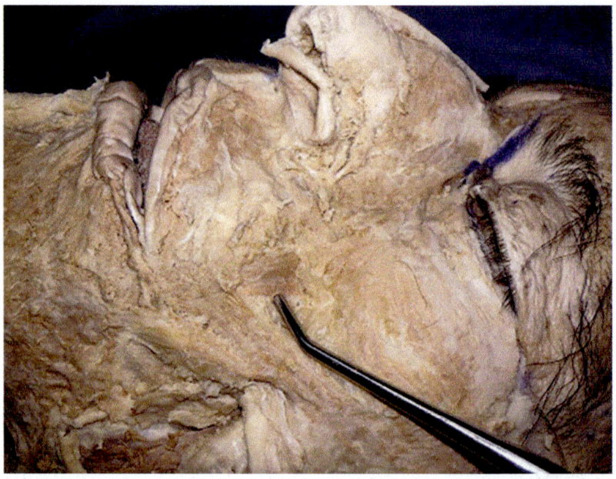

Fig. 3.51 With superficial fat layer and SMAS removed, a portion of the levator labii superioris (pointer) is seen traveling towards its insertion on the orbicularis oris muscle from its origin at the maxillary bone, along the inferior orbital rim

4. Starting over the zygoma, with a combination of sharp dissection with a # 15 blade (Fig. 3.48) and blunt dissection with spreading scissors (Fig. 3.49), dissect the fat from the underlying SMAS and orbital orbicularis muscle, toward the nasojugal fold. The SMAS will be studied in more detail in the "musculature" section below.
5. Care is taken to avoid going too deep into orbicularis muscle or too thin to avoid "button –holes" in this subcutaneous fatty layer.
6. As the dissection continues below, note that the subcutaneous fat is firmly attached to the orbicularis muscle at the orbital rim and parotid area, but more loosely attached in the region of the nasojugal and nasolabial folds as well as over the mandible.
7. Carry the sub-fat dissection inferiorly at the nasojugal and nasolabial area toward the oral commissure (Fig. 3.50).
8. Note the looser attachments in this area to the underlying Levator Labii Superioris muscle (Fig. 3.51) and Levator Labii Superioris Alaeque Nasi Muscle (Fig. 3.52).
9. At the inferior orbital rim, continue the sub-fat dissection inferiorly toward the mandible and laterally to the parotid gland (Fig. 3.53), exposing the underlying Zygomatic Minor

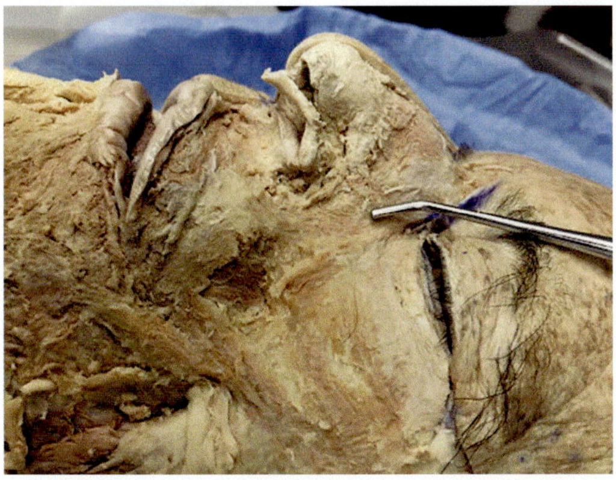

Fig. 3.52 With superficial fat layer and SMAS removed, the levator labii superioris alaeque nasi (pointer) is seen originating from the maxillary bone, then extends inferiorly to insert into the skin along the ala of the nose and the upper lip

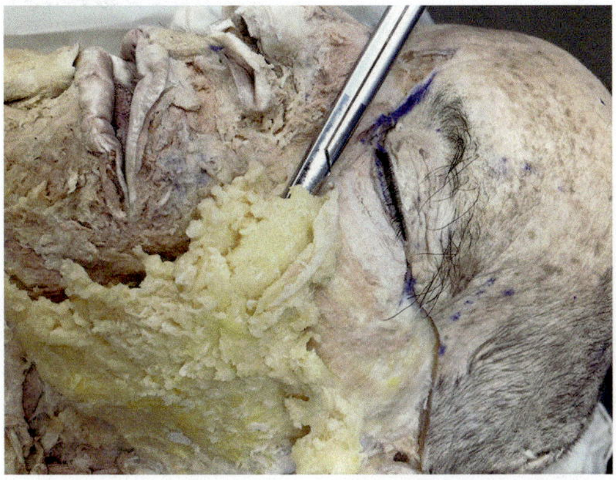

Fig. 3.53 Sub-fat and SMAS dissection inferiorly toward mandible and laterally toward parotid gland

muscle and Zygomatic Major muscle (Fig. 3.54).

10. At the oral commissure, continue the subcutaneous fat dissection laterally over the mandible (Fig. 3.55). Note the looser attachments in this area.
11. Identify the superior and inferior jowl fat pads (Fig. 3.55).
12. Expose and identify the underlying Risorius muscle, and orbicularis oris muscle (Fig. 3.56).
13. Below the oral commissure, identify the mentalis muscle, depressor labii oris muscle, and the depressor anguli oris muscle (Fig. 3.57).

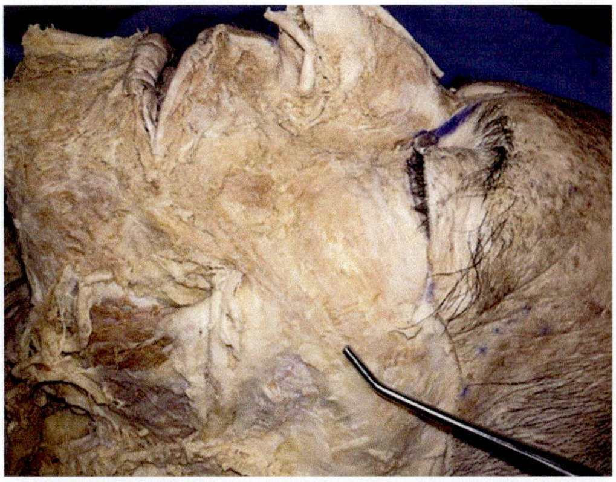

Fig. 3.54 With the superficial fat and SMAS removed, the zygomaticus major (left of pointer) and zygomatic minor (right of pointer) are demonstrated

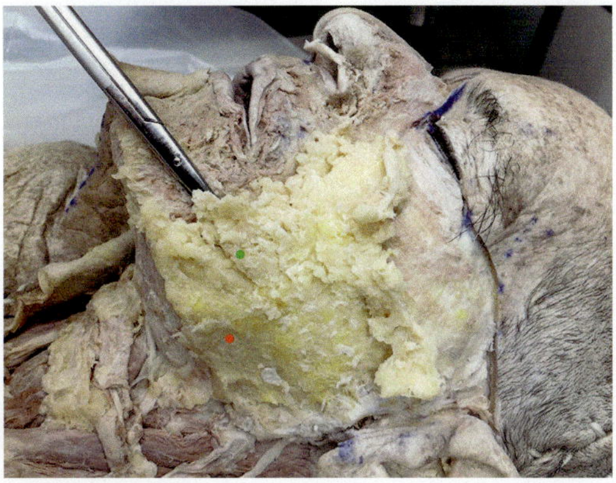

Fig. 3.55 Dissection over mandible. Note the continuity of the superior jowl fat (green dot) and inferior jowl fat (red dot) with the superficial malar fat pads

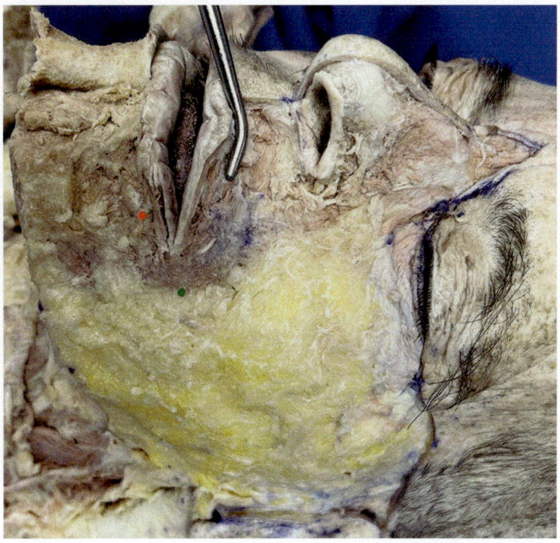

Fig. 3.56 Orbicularis oris muscle. Note fibers of upper lip (pointer) and lower lip (red dot) and beginning of the risorius muscle (green dot)

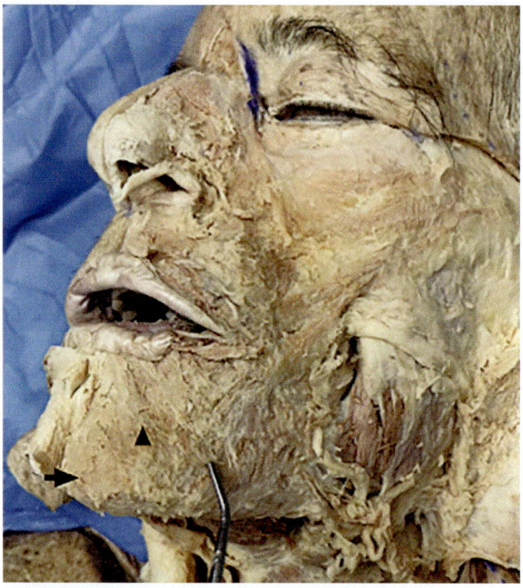

Fig. 3.57 The inferior perioral musculature is shown, to include the mentalis (arrow), the depressor labii inferioris (triangle), as well as the depressor anguli oris displayed with the probe

Musculature

The muscles of the midface and lower face are divided into two layers: (1) the superficial muscles of facial expression (Fig. 3.58) and (2) the deep muscles of mastication (Fig. 3.59).

Superficial Musculoaponeurotic System (SMAS)

Deep to the dermis and subcutaneous fat, a fibromuscular sheath is found encasing the superficial muscles of facial expression as well as the parotid gland, branches of the facial nerve (CN VII), and branches of the facial artery and vein. This fibromuscular superficial facial sheath is known as the superficial musculoaponeurotic system (SMAS). The SMAS varies in thickness, being thickest over the parotid gland and thinnest as it extends medially toward the nasalis muscle. Fine subcu-

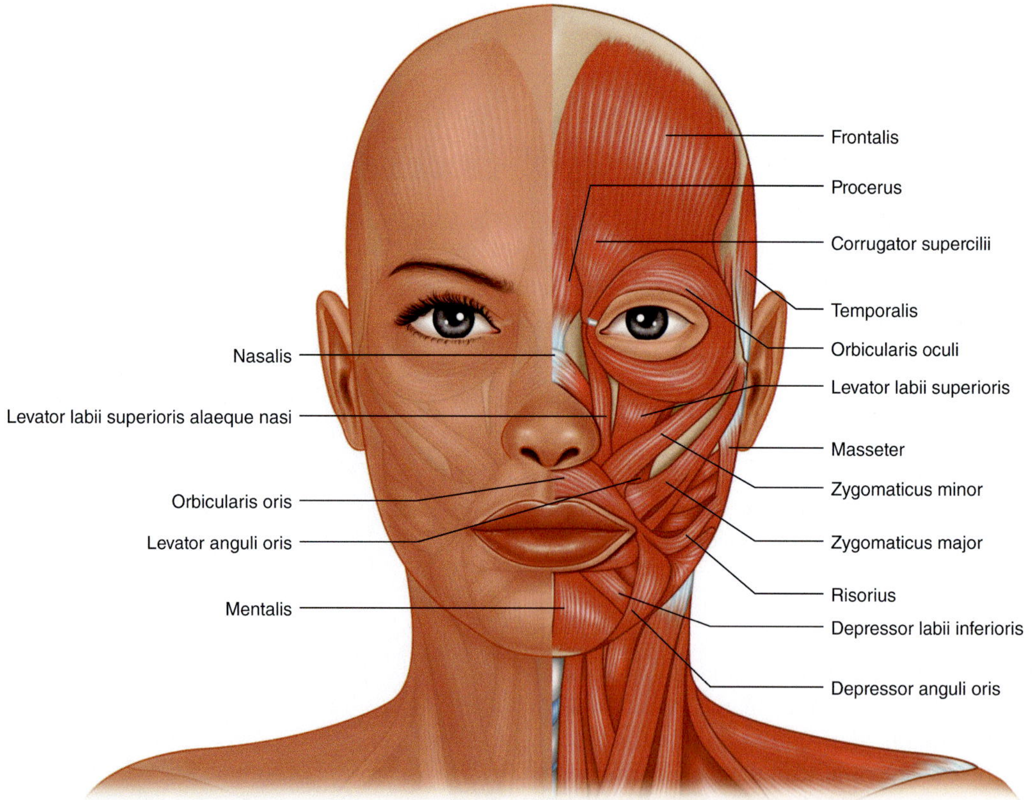

Fig. 3.58 Superficial muscles of the face (muscles of facial expression)

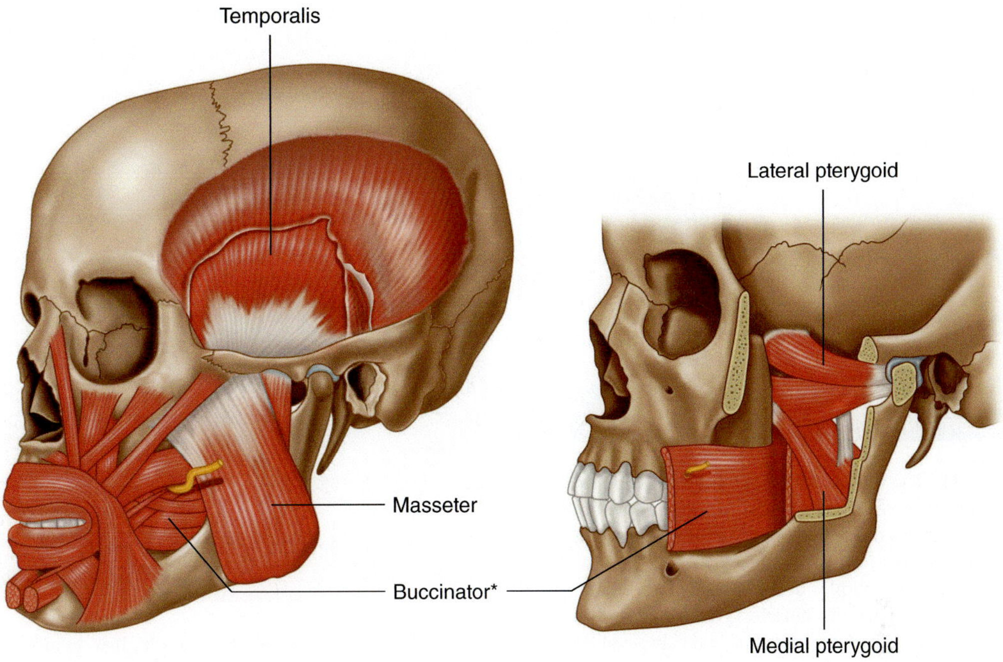

Fig. 3.59 Deep muscles of the face (muscles of mastication)

taneous reticular attachments of the SMAS to the overlying dermis and subcutaneous fat were severed above, during the subcutaneous dissection and during the subcutaneous superficial fat dissection. Posteriorly, the SMAS overlies the facial musculature and is anchored to the periosteum at only a few locations, by true retaining ligaments.

Clinical Correlation

The facial mimetic muscles are essential for facial expression, eyelid function, and for speech. These subcutaneous reticular attachments from the SMAS to the dermis translate facial expression to the skin of the entire face and neck. With age, these retinacular fibers attenuate leading to prolapse of subcutaneous tissue and the development of the malar, nasojugal, nasolabial, and mesolabial folds.

1. With further blunt dissection and reflection of the sub subcutaneous superficial fat layer, expose the underlying SMAS (Figs. 3.60 and 3.61).

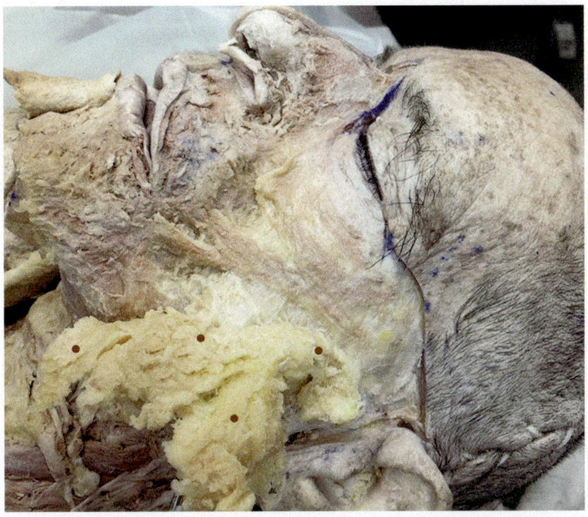

Fig. 3.60 Laterally reflected subcutaneous fat and SMAS (brown dots), exposing underlying facial musculature

2. Superotemporally, identify the SMAS joining with temporoparietal fascia near the frontozygomatic suture. These firm attachments mark the superior anatomical end of the SMAS in the face. Above this, the temporoparietal fascia continues to invest the frontalis as the SMAS in the forehead (*see* Section "The Superficial Temporalis Fascia" in Chap. 2).

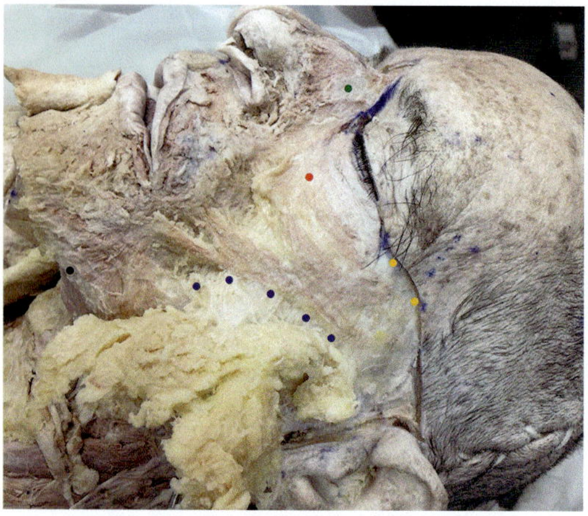

Fig. 3.61 The reflected SMAS joins the temporoparietal fascia near the frontozygomatic suture (yellow dots) and receives invested interdigitations of the orbicularis oculi beyond the inferior orbital rim (red dot), fuses with the parotid gland (purple dot). The SMAS thins as it approaches the nasalis muscle (green dot) and prior to reflection, fuses with the platysma at the angle of the mandible (black dot)

3. Superomedially, identify the SMAS investing the orbicularis oculi beyond the inferior orbital rim.
4. Laterally, identify the SMAS fusing with the fascia of the parotid gland.
5. Medially, note how the SMAS slowly thins as it approaches the nasalis muscle.
6. Inferiorly, the SMAS is continuous with the platysma at the angle of the mandible. Recall that the platysma muscle forms a sheet of muscle covering the anterior neck. Its inferior attachment is the superficial fascia of the upper thorax.

Periocular Musculature

For a detailed dissection of the eyelid, see *Surgical Anatomy of the Eyelids, Orbit, and Lacrimal System: A Dissection Manual*, Chap. 2.

1. Identify *the orbicularis oculi muscle* (Fig. 3.62) originating from the medial orbital margin. It is arbitrarily divided into the pretarsal, preseptal, and orbital components. Anatomically, only the orbital portion of the orbicularis oculi muscles of the lower lid is considered part of the midface.
2. Identify the pretarsal orbicularis oculi as it is firmly attached to the anterior surface of the tarsus. Note how it extends toward the lateral orbital tubercle of Whitnall, within the lateral orbital rim.
3. Note how the preseptal and orbital components insert into the lateral palpebral raphe on the zygoma.

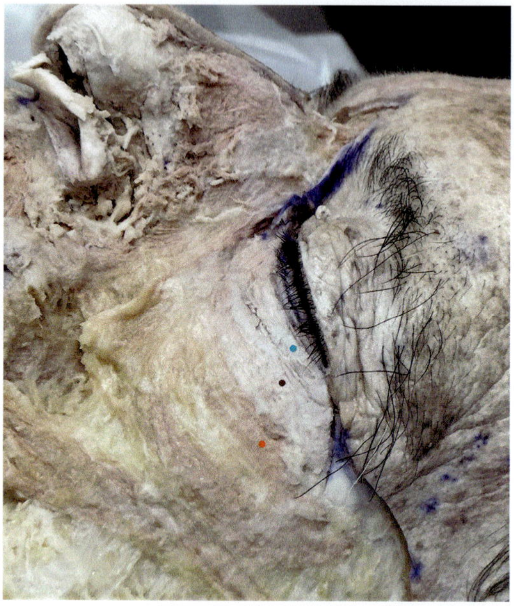

Fig. 3.62 The orbicularis oculi muscle. It is divided into the pretarsal (blue dot), preseptal (brown dot), and orbital (orange dot) components. Note how the orbital portion of the orbicularis oculi muscles is in continuum with the midface

Clinical Correlation

The orbicularis oculi muscle functions as a protractor of the eyelid. The finer pretarsal fibers are used for reflex blinking. Both the pretarasal and preseptal fibers are engaged in voluntary blinking of the eyelid. Forceful closure, such as winking recruits the larger orbital component. The orbital component extends beyond the inferior orbital rim, and via the SMAS is continuous with the other facial muscles in this plane.

Midfacial Musculature

Five facial muscles of expression within the SMAS elevate the lip and oral commissure (Figs. 3.58 and 3.63).

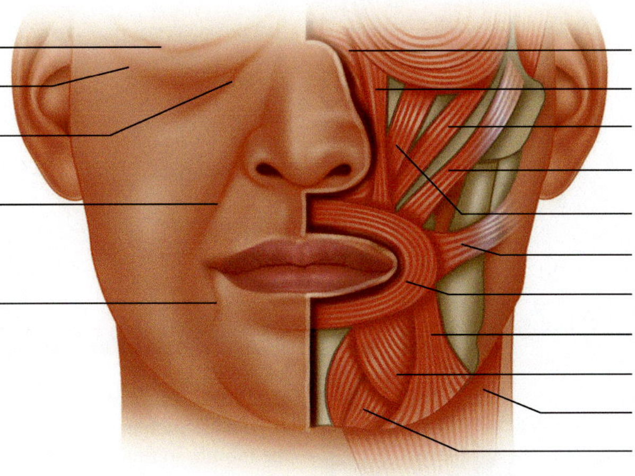

Fig. 3.63 SMAS components that elevate the lip and oral commissure and associated skin creases

Clinical Correlation

The simultaneous action of these five muscles, as listed below, functions to elevate the cheeks, chin, lips, and oral commissures, assisting with the creation of the nasolabial folds.

1. Identify the *levator labii superioris* (Fig. 3.51) It originates below the medial infraorbital rim, extending inferiorly from the orbital orbicularis oculi muscle, to cover the infraorbital foramen and eventually blends with the orbicularis oris at the lateral lip. It functions to elevate the lip in a mostly vertical direction.
2. Identify the *levator labii superioris alaeque nasi* (Fig. 3.52). It originates from the upper frontal process of the maxilla, courses inferiorly along the side of the nose. It then splits into a wider medial head which inserts onto the skin of the lateral nostril and a narrower lateral head which inserts onto the skin of the upper lip. It functions to both flare the nostril and elevate the lip.
3. Identify the *levator anguli oris* (Figs. 3.58 and 3.64) It originates from the maxilla, approximately 1 cm inferior to the infraorbital foramen and inserts on the outer edge of the lip and modiolus. Identify the modiolus (Figs. 3.64 and 3.65) which is a point lateral to the angle of the mouth where several muscles of facial expression converge.
4. Identify the *zygomaticus major* muscle (Figs. 3.54 and 3.66). It originates at the zygomatic arch and inserts at the modiolus near the mouth. It moves the lips laterally and vertically. It is the most laterally located muscle involved in lip elevation.

Clinical Correlation

Contraction of the zygomatius major muscle creates the characteristic dimples, which can be a prominent facial feature for some people.

5. Identify the *zygomaticus minor* (Figs. 3.54 and 3.67) originates from the maxillary process of the zygomatic bone and inserts near the lip, just lateral to the insertion of the levator labii superioris muscle.

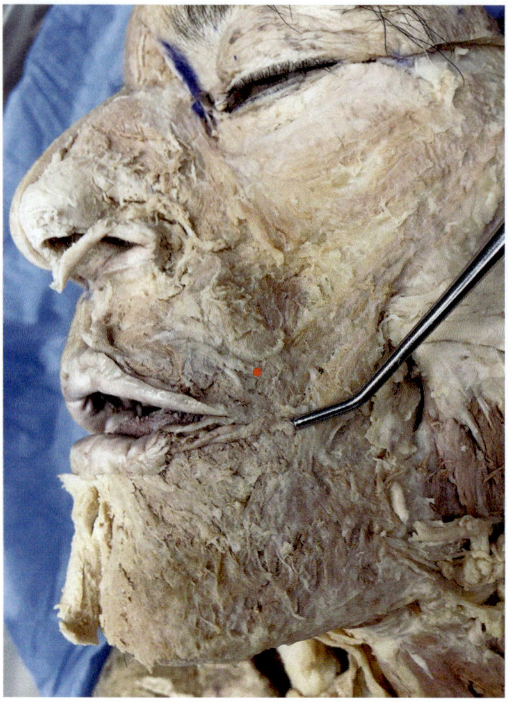

Fig. 3.64 The levator anguli oris (red dot), risorius muscle at tip of pointer and modiolus (posterior to pointer)

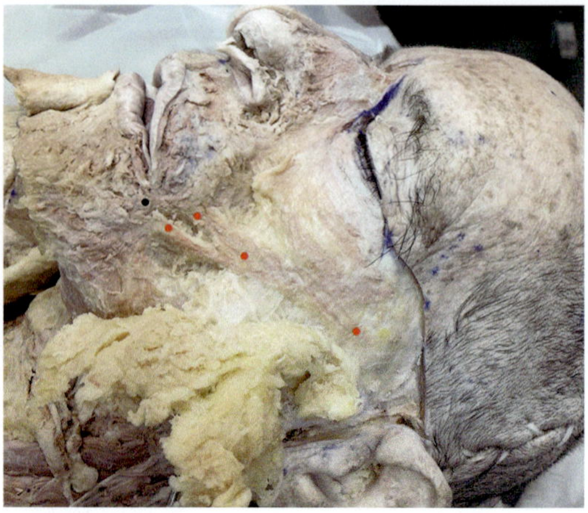

Fig. 3.66 Zygomaticus major muscle. It originates at the zygomatic arch and inserts at the modiolus (black dot) of the mouth. In this specimen, the muscle (red dots) is split by a fat pad

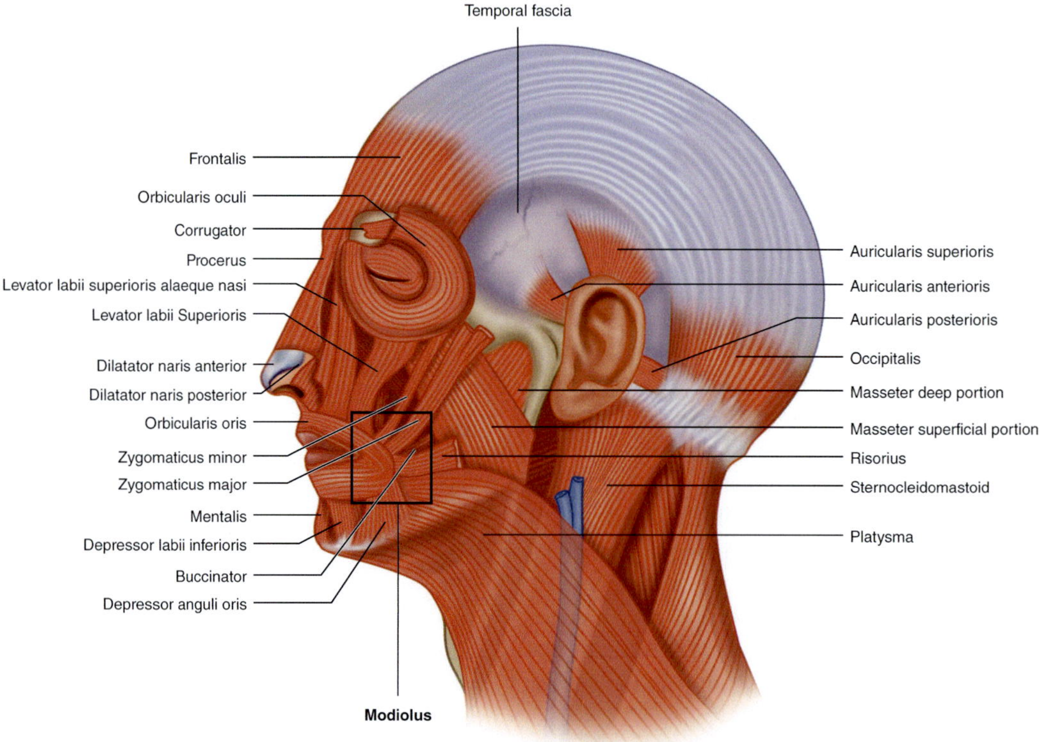

Fig. 3.65 Modiolus, a point lateral to the angle of the mouth where muscles of facial expression converge

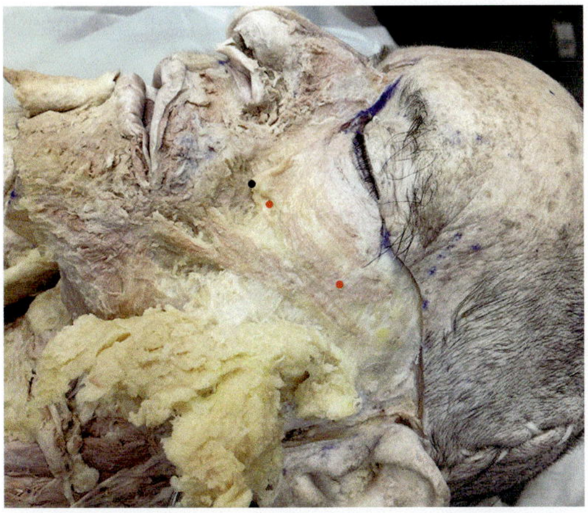

Fig. 3.67 Zygomaticus minor (red dots) originates from the maxillary process of the zygomatic bone and inserts near the lip, just lateral to the insertion of the levator labii superioris muscle (black dot)

Perioral Musculature

1. Expose *the orbicularis oris muscle* (Figs. 3.56 and 3.68). Note that the orbicularis oris fibers firmly insert directly onto the dermis around the mouth. These will be cut for better exposure.
2. Identify the superior and inferior portions of the orbicularis oris which surround the oral cavity. It is composed of muscle as well as fibrous membranes from other muscles inserting into the orbicularis oris.
3. Identify the origins of the orbicularis oris including the fibers of surrounding muscles including the buccinators, the nasal septum, and the area lateral to the incisive fossa of the mandible.

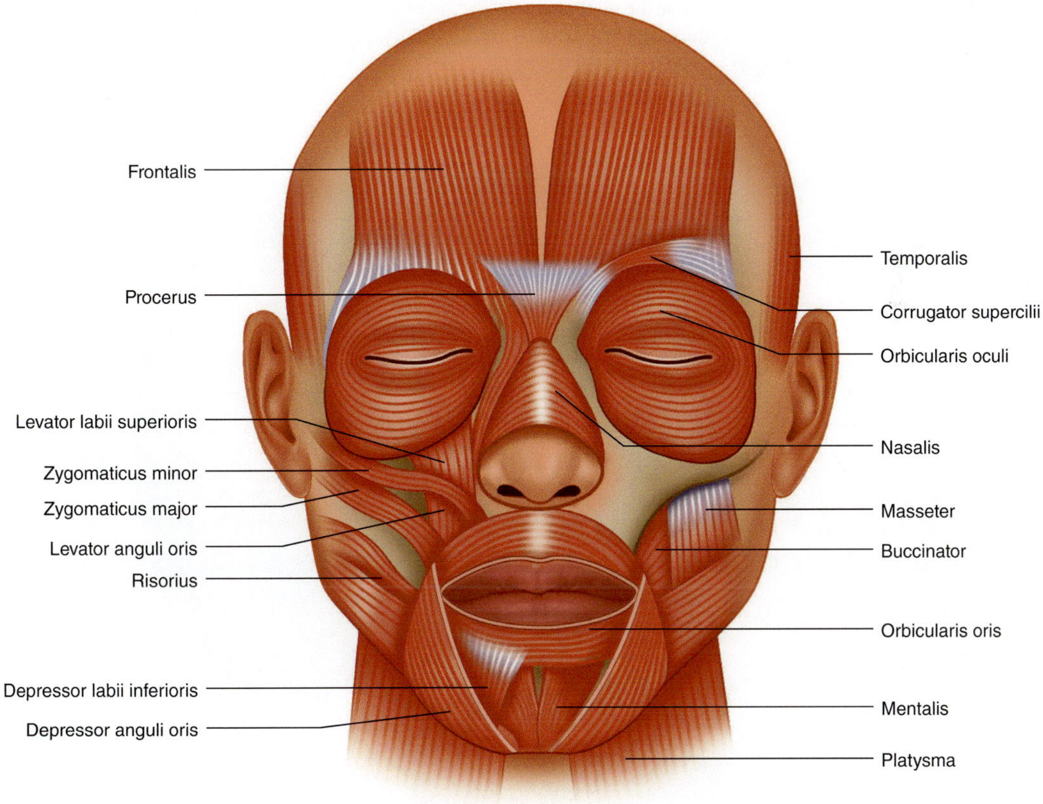

Fig. 3.68 Superficial facial and perioral musculature

4. Identify the *risorius muscle* (Fig. 3.69). It originates from the fascia of the masseter (Fig. 3.70) and inserts or fuses with the orbicularis oris at the corner of the mouth. Note how it lies just anterior to the lateral platysma fibers and pulls the corners of the mouth horizontally.
5. Identify further the modiolus, which is the point of confluence of the mimetic muscles near the oral commissure (*see* Fig. 3.65 and Fig. 3.66).
6. Within the oral cavity, palpate the thickness of the *buccinator muscle* (Fig. 3.71) lining the cheek. A deeper dissection is necessary as it lies deep to the muscles of the facial expression and will be done later in the dissection (Section "Buccinator Muscle").

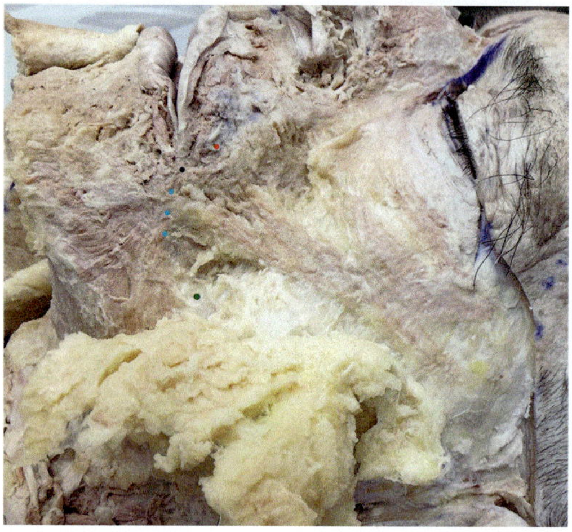

Fig. 3.69 Risorius muscle (blue dots). Note the modiolus (black dot), levator anguli oris (red dot), and fascia of deeper masseter muscle (green dot)

Clinical correlation

The buccinator muscle assists with the actions of sucking, blowing, and whistling to bring in or expel air from the oral cavity. Additionally, it contributes with mastication by providing tension to hold food between the cheeks and teeth.

Fig. 3.70 Masseter muscle and temporalis muscle

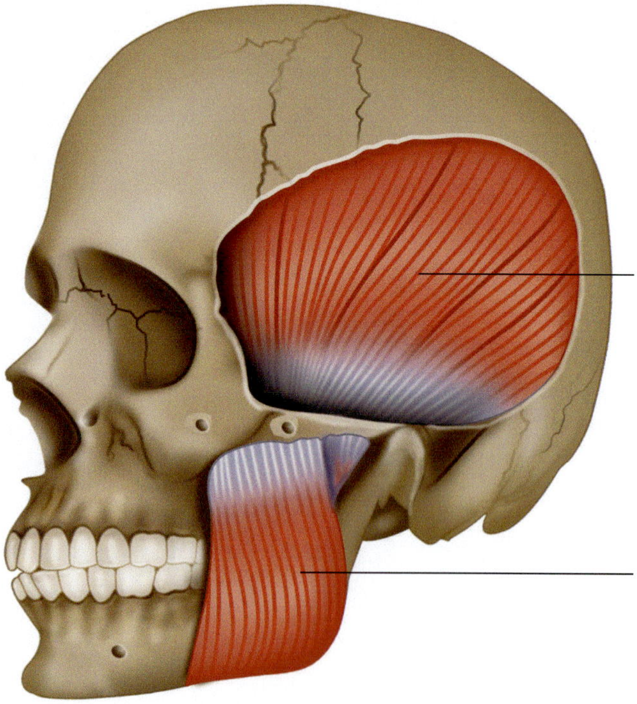

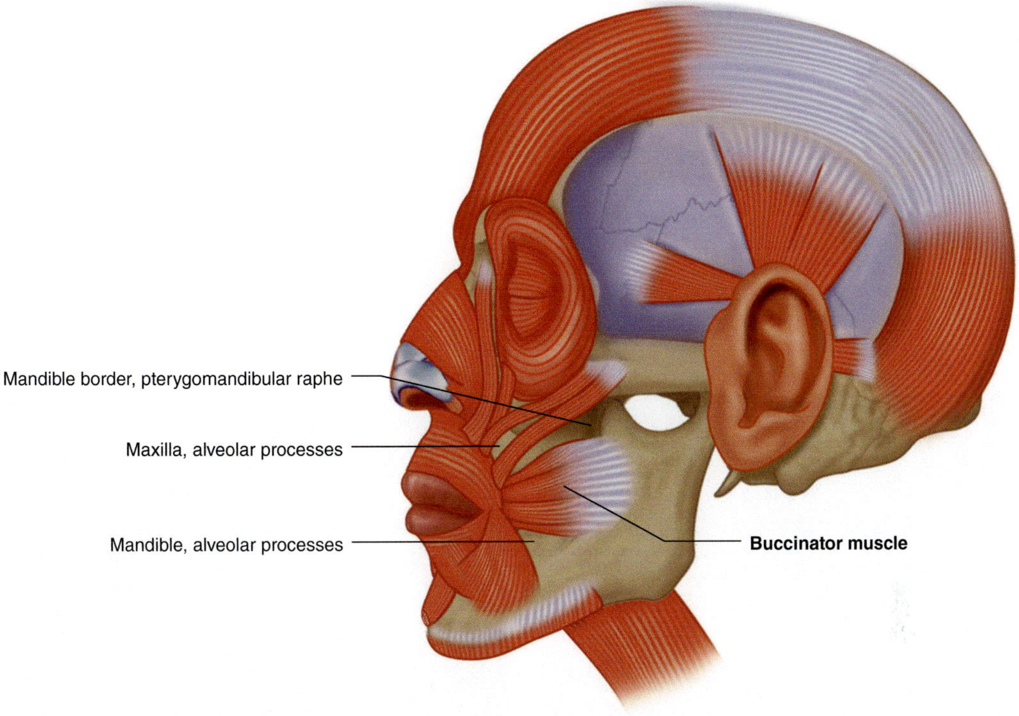

Fig. 3.71 Buccinator muscle. It arises anteriorly from the outer surfaces of the alveolar processes of the maxilla and mandible, and posteriorly from the anterior border of the pterygomandibular raphe

Sub-SMAS Dissection

Before proceeding with the sub-SMAS dissection, review and identify the anatomy of the of retaining ligaments and loose alveolar tissue described below. They will be sacrificed with further sub-SMAS dissection.

Retaining Ligaments

Numerous descriptions have been provided for the nomenclature of the facial ligamentous structure. In general, the facial ligaments can be divided into 1. supporting ligaments or reticular fibers extending superficially from the SMAS to the subcutaneous tissue and 2. true retaining ligaments which attach the superficial facial tissues deeply to the bone (Fig. 3.72).

The "retaining ligaments" include the orbitomalar ligament, the zygomatico-cutaneous ligament, and the masseteric cutaneous ligament.

Clinical Correlation

The true retaining ligaments are locations where the SMAS is firmly attached to either periosteum or the parotid fascia. These ligaments "anchor" the SMAS and skin in place and are the only structures restricting facial movement, thus limiting the glide planes of the face, making it prone to the effects of gravity.

1. Identify the *Orbitomalar Ligament*: It arises from the inferior orbital rim, travels superficially through the SMAS encasing the orbicularis oculi, passes through the subcutaneous fat, to insert onto the dermis in a "fan-like" fashion (Fig. 3.73). The dermal attachments were cut during the subcutaneous skin dissection above.

   It is firmly attached deeply to the periosteum of the maxillary bone at the inferior and lateral orbital rim (Fig. 3.74). The orbitomalar ligament

Fig. 3.72 The retaining ligaments

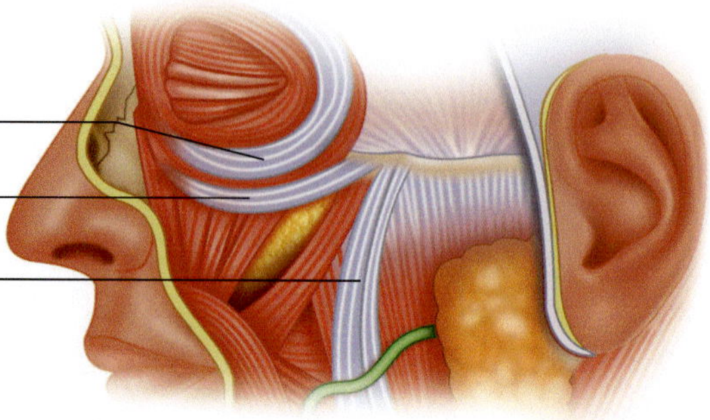

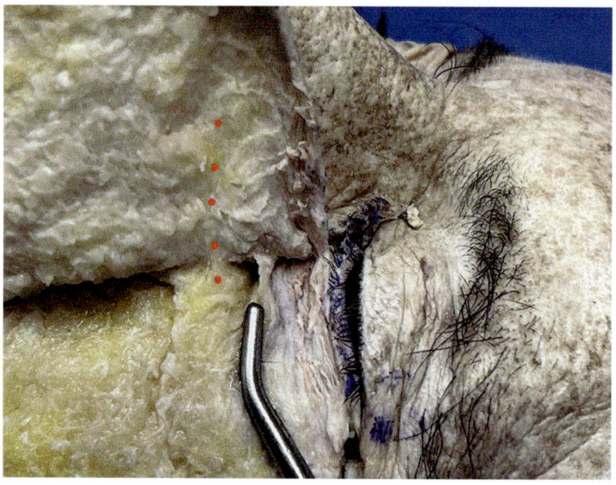

Fig. 3.73 Fan-like sub-dermal insertions of the Orbitomalar Ligament (red dots). Note the subcutaneous attachments at the nasojugal fold (pointer)

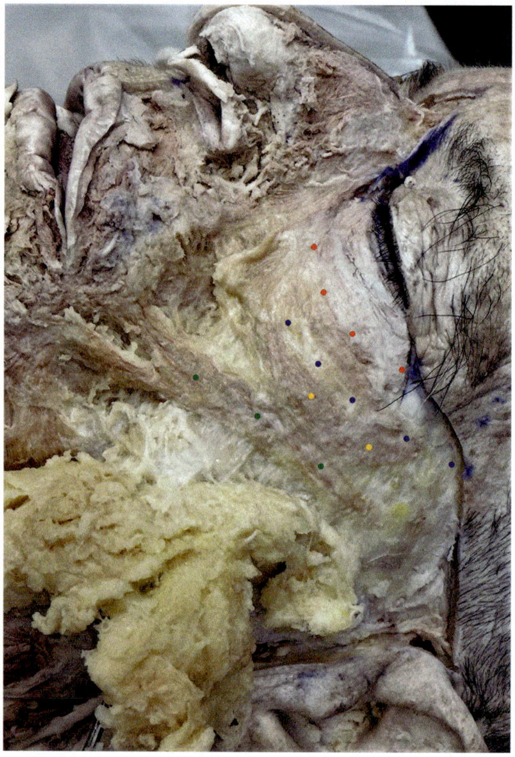

Fig. 3.74 The location of the orbitomalar ligament (red dots) and, the Zygomatico-Cutaneous Ligament (purple dots). Note the zygomaticus minor muscle (yellow dots), and the zygomaticus major muscle (green dots). The subcutaneous fat layer is reflected laterally

extends from 5 mm lateral to the lateral orbital rim toward the nasojugal fold overlying the anterior lacrimal crest. Note how it is strongest laterally.

Clinical Correlation

The orbitomalar ligament suspends the subcutaneous tissue and skin onto the malar eminence (Fig. 3.75). With age, the orbitomalar ligament and skin lose elasticity causing the SOOF and sub-SMAS deep fat to descend. As a result, the orbital rim, nasojugal and malar folds becomes more prominent. Additionally, the orbital septum attenuates, allowing the post septal orbital fat to prolapse creating the appearance of "bags" under the eye. Resuspension of this ligament and fat management restore the midface anatomy to its youthful position

2. Identify the *Zygomatico-Cutaneous Ligament (Zygomatic ligament/McGregor's Patch).*

It is a firm attachment of the SMAS on the zygomatic bone, lateral to the origin of the zygomaticus major muscle, approximately 45 mm anterior to the tragus (Figs. 3.76 and 3.77). Trace this curvilinear ligament, as it

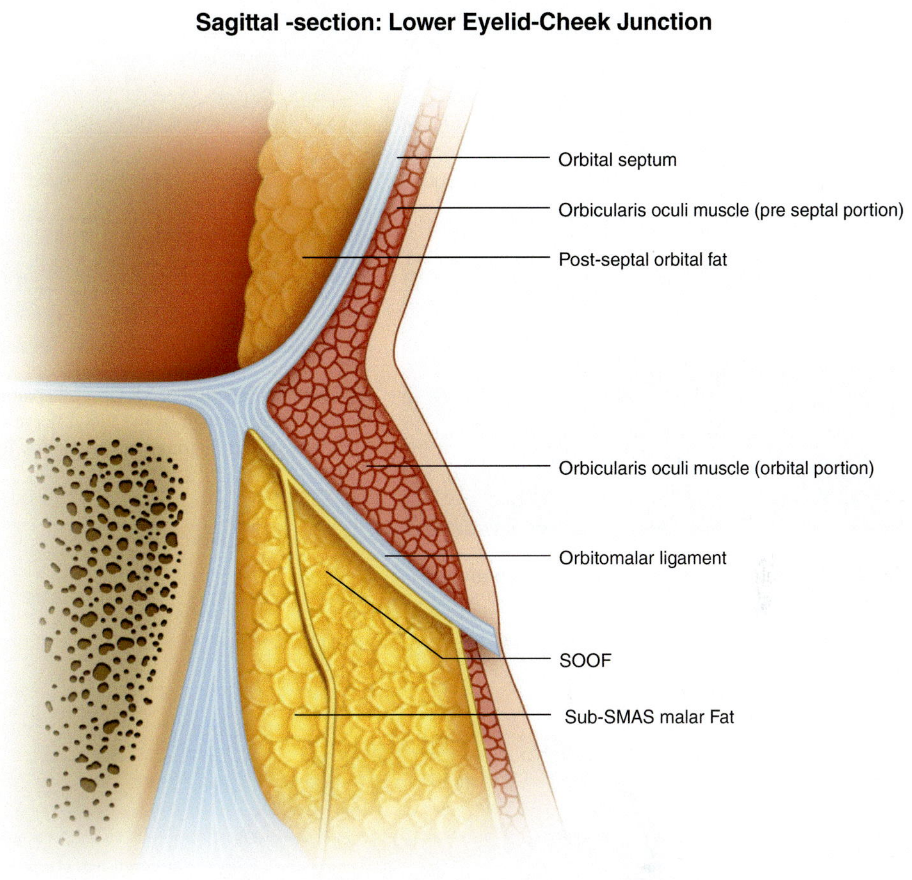

Fig. 3.75 Sagittal-section of the Orbitomalar-retaining ligament, suspending the SOOF and deep fat pads in the infraorbital area

extends anteriorly and medially above the origin of the zygomaticus minor to the inferior border of the zygoma. The average width is approximated to be 14.5 mm.

Clinical Correlation
(McGregor's Patch) is often used synonymously with the zygomatic cutaneous ligament. The patch is composed of the zygomatic ligaments as well as the masseteric ligaments. The clinical importance of this "patch" is to signify the close proximity of a perforating branch of the transverse facial artery (Figs. 3.78 and 3.79), the parotid fascia, and zygomatic branches of the facial nerve. Its careful release is necessary to facilitate mobilization of the overlying soft tissue for aesthetic manipulation.

3. Identify the *Masseteric Cutaneous Ligaments*.
4. Superficial fibers may have been cut in the earlier subcutaneous dissection as they extend through the SMAS to attach to the dermis. They begin approximately 42 mm anterior to the tragus (Fig. 3.80) and end 25 mm posterior to the superoanterior edge of the masseter. (Fig. 3.81).

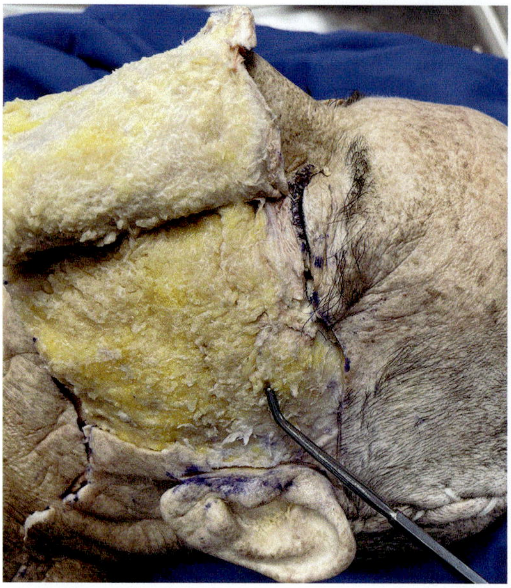

Fig. 3.76 Location of McGregor's patch deep to the lateral superficial malar fat pad

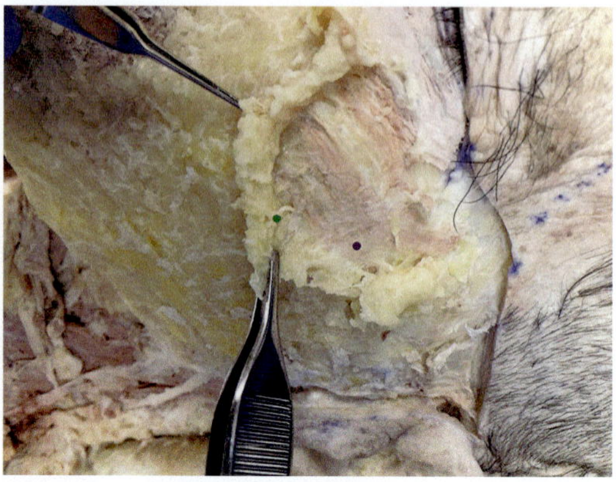

Fig. 3.77 Dissection of McGregor's patch demonstrating the zygomatic branch of the facial nerve (green dot), and a portion of the zygomatico-cutaneous ligament (purple dot)

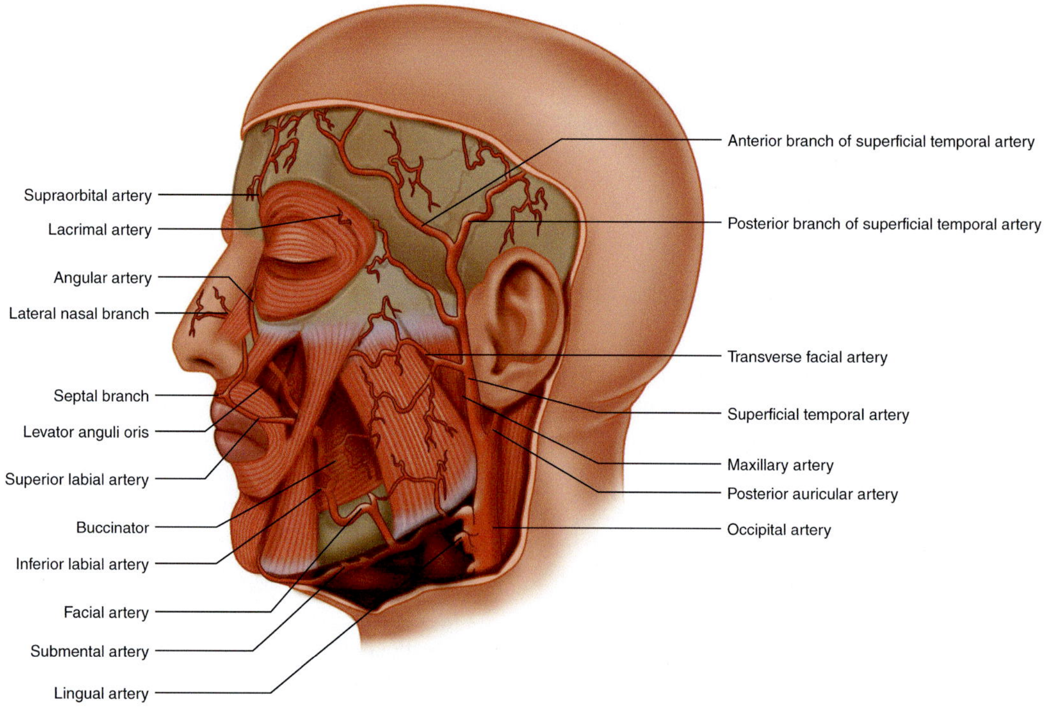

Fig. 3.78 Arterial supply to the face

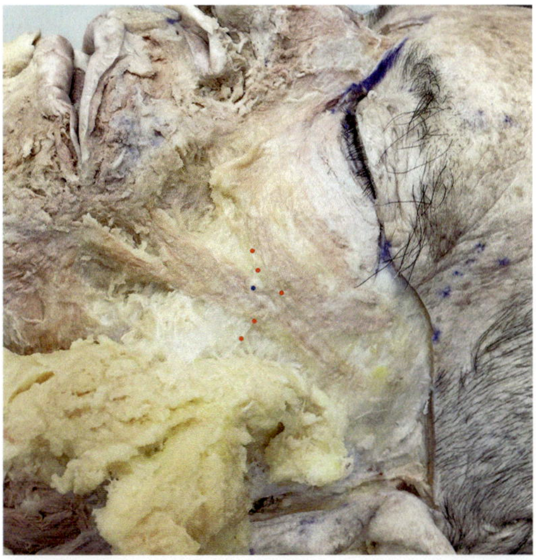

Fig. 3.79 Transverse facial artery (blue dot) and zygomatic branches of the facial nerve (red dots)

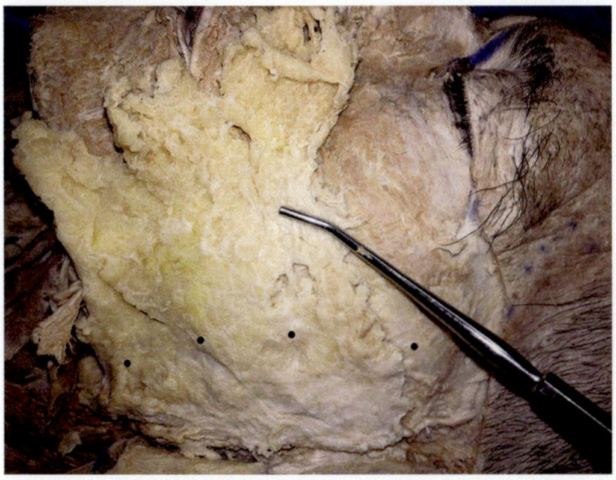

Fig. 3.80 Location of the Masseteric cutaneous ligament (black dots). Pointer overlies the subcutaneous fat

5. Note how the ligament extends superiorly almost to the zygomatic arch and extends inferiorly beyond the mandibular edge.

> **Clinical Correlation**
> These tight attachments to the midface skin are usually severed during midface lift in order to elevate the skin to its youthful position.

Loose Areolar Tissue

1. As dissection continues into the lower cheek, notice that a less adherent sub-SMAS areolar plane exists, directly overlying the masseter muscle and also deep to the platsyma in the neck (*see* Chap. 4).

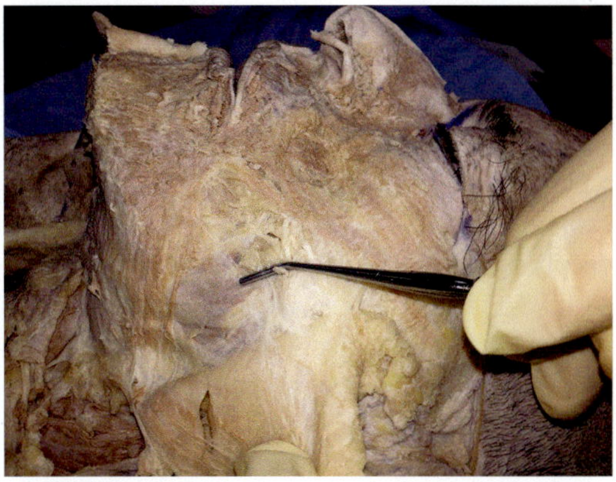

Fig. 3.81 Deep to the SMAS, emanating from the anterior aspect of the masseter muscle (tip of pointer) is the masseteric cutaneous ligament (under the pointer)

> **Clinical Correlation**
> The loose areolar tissue is located between the retaining ligaments and allows the superficial layers of the face (SMAS) to move smoothly over the deep tissues (deep fascia and periosteum). These planes are referred to as "glide planes." These glide planes enlarge or stretch with age due to laxity of the retaining ligaments and contribute to descent of the skin and soft tissue of the face.

2. The sub-SMAS plane is quite avascular except for a perforating branch of the transverse facial artery which travels within McGregor's patch.

> **Clinical Correlation**
> Blood vessels and nerves do not enter the glide planes. Therefore, these planes are safe surgical planes of dissection, without risk of bleeding or disruption of innervation.

3. The facial artery also travels in the deep plane and is located along the mandible and in a superior and medial direction. It will be studied later in this dissection (Section "The Facial artery").

Sub-SMAS Dissection

As stated above, the fibers of the muscles of facial expression interdigitate within the SMAS which are not only attached superficially to the skin as noted above, but they are also attached deeply by the facial ligamentous system.

1. Next carefully incise, then dissect in the submuscular plane starting in the malar region (Fig. 3.82).
2. Continue the submuscular malar dissection anteriorly and superiorly to the inferior border of the orbicularis oculi, transecting the thick zygomatic cutaneous ligament of the malar fat pad (McGregor's patch).
3. Carry the dissection medially under the zygomaticus muscles toward the nasojugal fold (Figs. 3.83 and 3.84).
4. Cut the orbicularis muscle at the lid margin to allow for mobilization of the plane medially (Fig. 3.85).

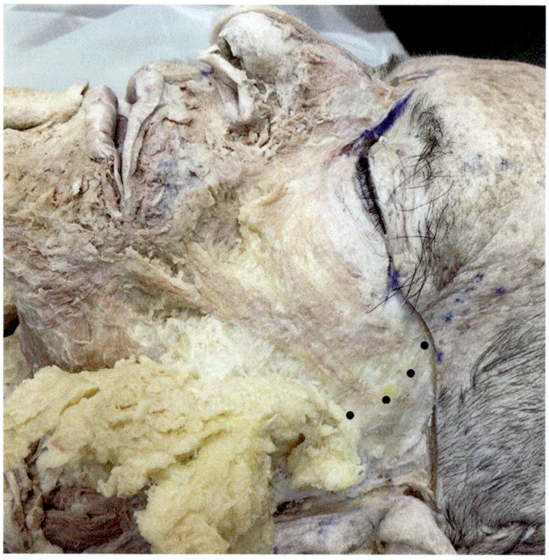

Fig. 3.82 Black dots indicate site of incision into the muscles of facial expression, in malar region

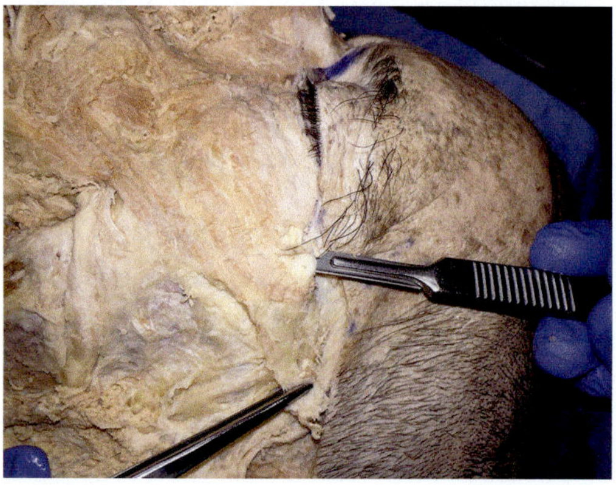

Fig. 3.83 Submuscular dissection in the malar region is initiated in the region of the zygomaticus muscles and carried medially

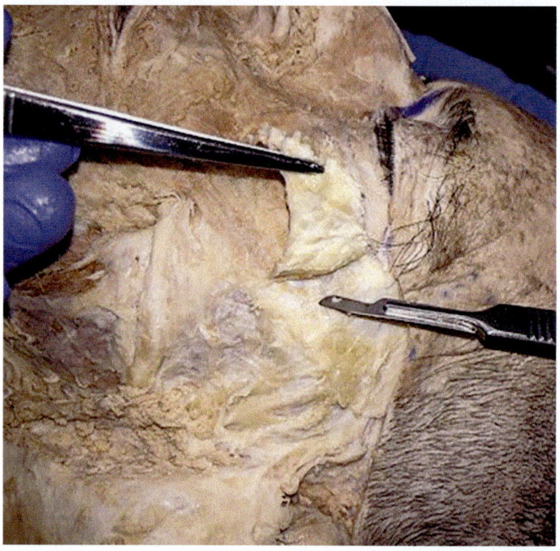

Fig. 3.84 Submuscular dissection in the malar region

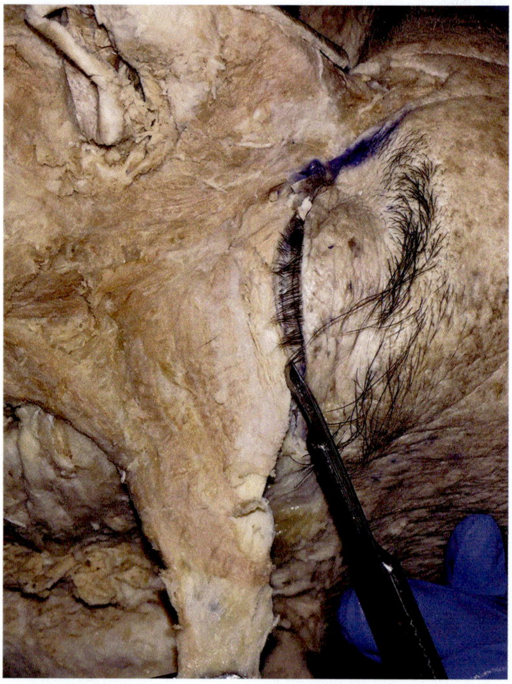

Fig. 3.85 Release of pre-tarsal orbicularis muscle at the lid margin to allow for medial reflection of facial musculature

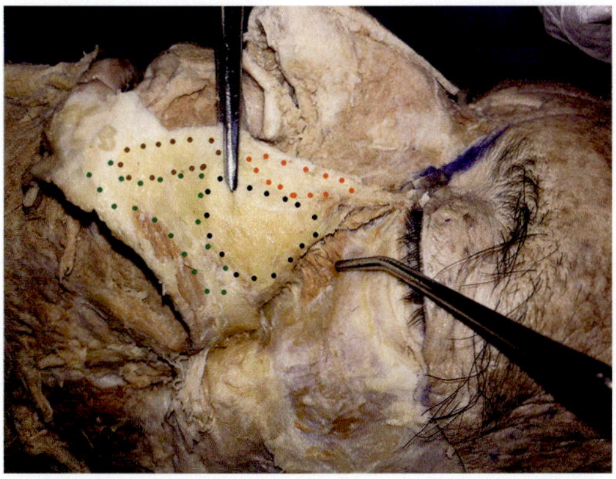

Fig. 3.86 The levator labii superioris (pointer) near its origin from the maxillary bone, along the inferior orbital rim. Note how the medial SOOF (orange dots), and lateral SOOF (brown dots), are adjacent to the sub-SMAS malar fat (black dots) and sub-SMAS lateral fat (green)

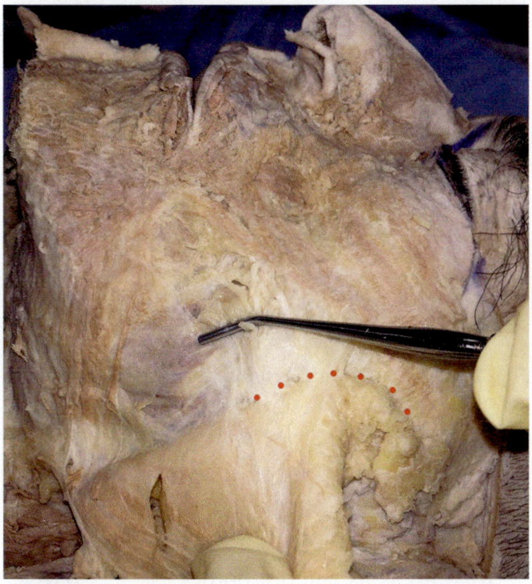

Fig. 3.87 Site of parotid fascial incision overlying the gland (red dots). Pointer on masseter muscle

5. Continue the dissection medially exposing a portion of the levator labii superioris (Fig. 3.86) near its origin at the maxillary bone, along the medial inferior orbital rim. Note how it extends inferiorly from the orbital orbicularis oculi muscle.
6. Also note how the levator labii superioris covers the infraorbital foramen and eventually blends with the orbicularis oris at the lateral lip.
7. With sharp dissection carry the incision inferiorly in front of the ear and anterior border of the parotid gland (Fig. 3.87). Caution is taken to avoid deep dissection into the parotid gland. The parotid gland and duct will be further dissected below.

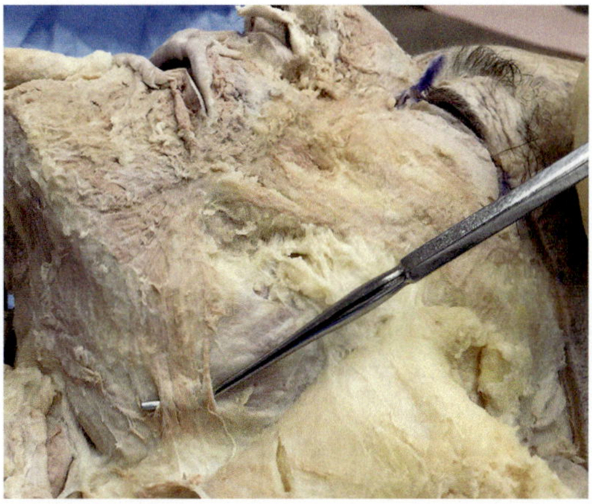

Fig. 3.88 Sub-SMAS dissection of lateral platysma muscle fibers (pointer) at lateral aspect of mandible

8. Continue the dissection toward the posterior border of the platysma (Fig. 3.88) just inferior to the angle of the mandible.

Deep Muscles and Structures of the Face

Muscles of Mastication

The muscles of mastication (*see* Fig. 3.59) are a group of muscles that are involved in chewing. They lie within the deep fascia that lines the maxillary bone of the midface and give support for the more superficial facial layers.

They consist of the 1. *temporalis muscle*, 2. *medial pterygoid muscle*, 3. *lateral pterygoid muscle*, 4. *masseter muscle*, and 5. *buccinator muscle* which is sometimes referred to as an accessory muscle of mastication.

1. The temporalis muscle. The temporalis muscle was discussed in Chap. 2 (Section "Temporal dissection") of this manual. It originates on the temporal fossa of the temporal bone (*see* Fig. 3.70) and inserts on the coronoid process and anterior ramus of the mandible; it elevates and retracts the mandible.

The medial and lateral pterygoids lie in the infratemporal fossa (*see* Fig. 3.59) are mentioned below but will not be dissected. Below is a description of each:

2. Medial Pterygoid muscle.
   (a) It has two heads.
   (b) The deep head originates on the medial aspect of the lateral pterygoid process of the sphenoid and inserts on the medial surface of the angle and ramus of the mandible.
   (c) The superficial head originates on the tuberosity of the maxilla and inserts with the deep head on the mandibular angle.
   (d) The medial pterygoid elevates the mandible and moves it to the opposite side.
3. The lateral pterygoid.
   (a) It is triangular in shape and is at right angles to the medial head.
   (b) It also has two heads:
   (c) The upper head originates from the infratemporal fossa of the sphenoid and inserts on the temporomandibular joint capsule and mandible.
   (d) The lower head originates from the lateral surface of the lateral pterygoid plate and inserts with the upper head.
   (e) The lateral pterygoid protrudes the mandible anteriorly and moves it to the opposite side.

The dissection below will focus on the masseter muscle and buccinator muscles in the cheek area. Closely related structures of surgical importance including the parotid duct, facial nerve, and facial artery will also be dissected.

The Masseter Muscle

On the lateral aspect of the lower face near the angle of the mandible, the masseter muscle was identified above (*see* Fig. 3.70). It is a large muscle of mastication (not facial expression) and it is the strongest. The masseter moves the mandible posteriorly and superiorly.

1. Reflect the superficial fat and underlying SMAS layers laterally to expose the anterior border of the masseter muscle (*see* Fig. 3.87).

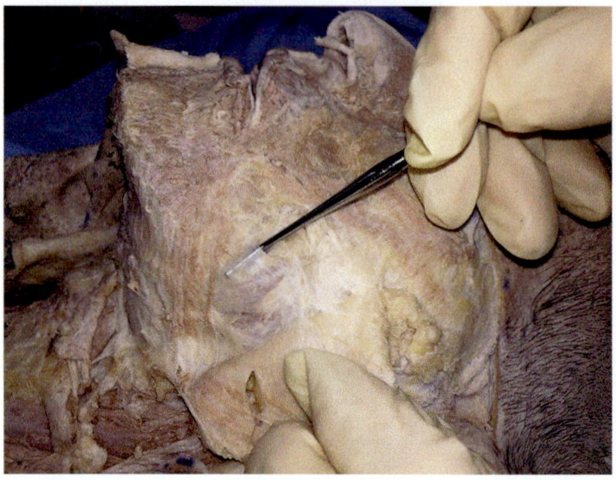

Fig. 3.89 Fibrous septae of the masseteric cutaneous ligaments at the anterior border of the masseter muscle

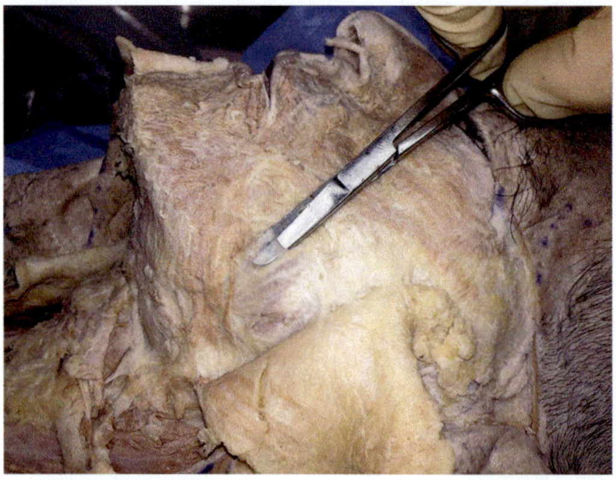

Fig. 3.90 Lysis of fibrous septae exposing anterior border of masseter muscle

2. Next elevate, bluntly by vertically spreading the scissors, from the anterior border of the parotid gland, over the masseter muscle as far forward as its anterior border.
3. Note the areolar plane overlying the masseter muscle.
4. The fibrous septae of the masseteric cutaneous ligaments are encountered, at the muscle's anterior border (Fig. 3.89).
5. With scissors or a 15 blade, cut the fibrous septae of the masseteric cutaneous ligaments (Fig. 3.90).
6. Now carry the dissection in the sub-platysmal plane anteriorly over the masseter border and inferiorly to the lower border of the mandible (Fig. 3.91). Care is taken to avoid cutting the facial artery in this location.

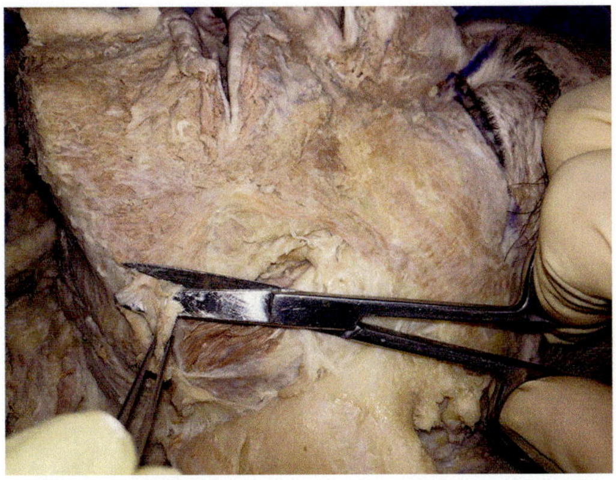

Fig. 3.91 Dissection over the masseter muscle at the lower border of the mandible, in region of the facial artery

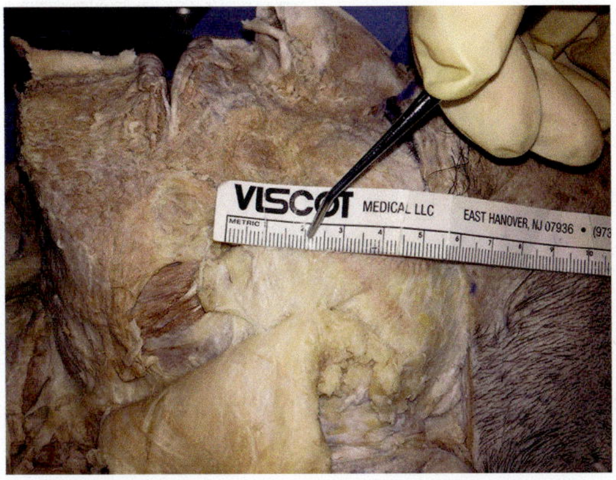

Fig. 3.92 Location of parotid duct 2 cm inferior to zygomatic arch

The Parotid Duct

1. Identify the *parotid duct* where it crosses the surface of the masseter muscle approximately 2 cm inferior to the zygomatic arch (Fig. 3.92). It is a relatively large structure about 2–3 mm in diameter.
2. Use blunt dissection to follow the parotid duct anteriorly past the anterior border of the masseter muscle where the duct turns medially into the cheek (Fig. 3.93).
3. With a probe or spreading scissors, bluntly dissect the parotid duct posteriorly thru buccal fat to the anterior margin of *the parotid gland* (Fig. 3.94). In some specimens an accessory parotid gland is present.
4. Further dissect the parotid duct anteriorly as it pierces the buccinator muscle (Fig. 3.95). Recall that it then drains into the oral cavity lateral to the second maxillary molar tooth.

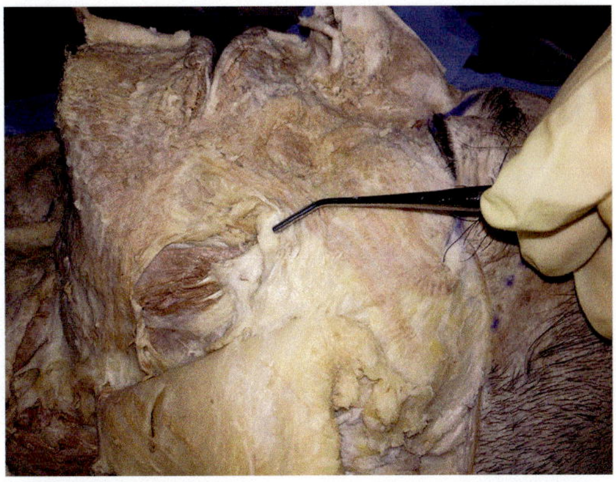

Fig. 3.93 Parotid duct

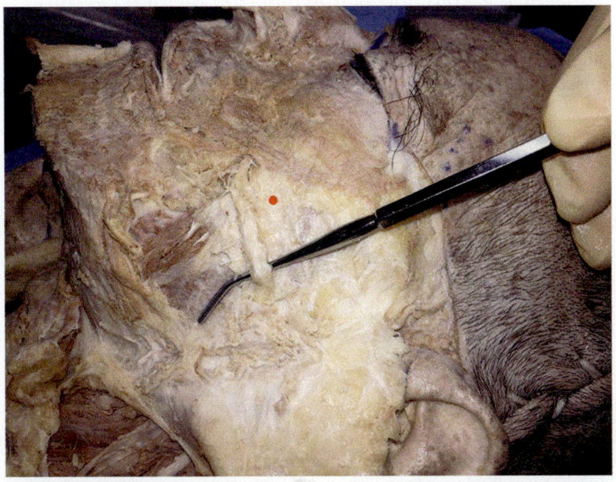

Fig. 3.94 Parotid duct exiting anterior margin of parotid gland. Note buccal fat (orange dot)

> **Clinical Correlation**
> Care is given with gingival nerve blocks to avoid the gingival opening of the parotid duct.

5. The parotid gland is enclosed within the parotid sheath which is continuous with the deep cervical fascia. With scissors or sharp dissection incise this layer (Fig. 3.96), exposing the parotid gland and branches of the facial nerve.

The Facial Nerve

1. Carefully dissect the multiple *buccal branches* of the facial nerve which course together superiorly or inferiorly, but parallel to the parotid duct (Fig. 3.97).

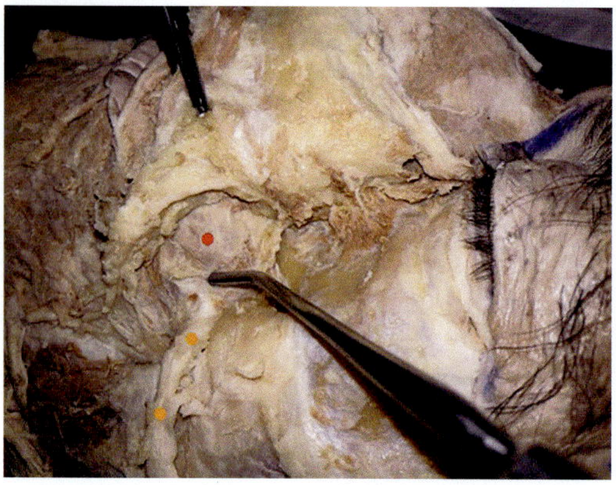

Fig. 3.95 Dissection carried medially, exposing the deep muscular plane. The probe delineates the medial extension of the parotid duct (yellow dots) piercing the buccinator muscle (red dot) before entering the oral cavity

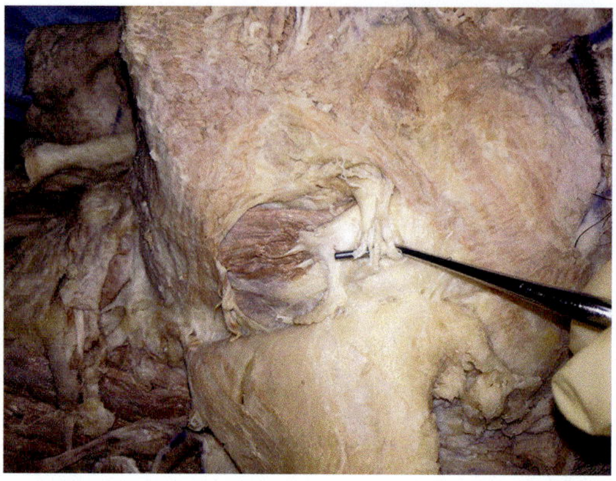

Fig. 3.97 Buccal branches of facial nerve. The tip of the pointer is on the parotid duct

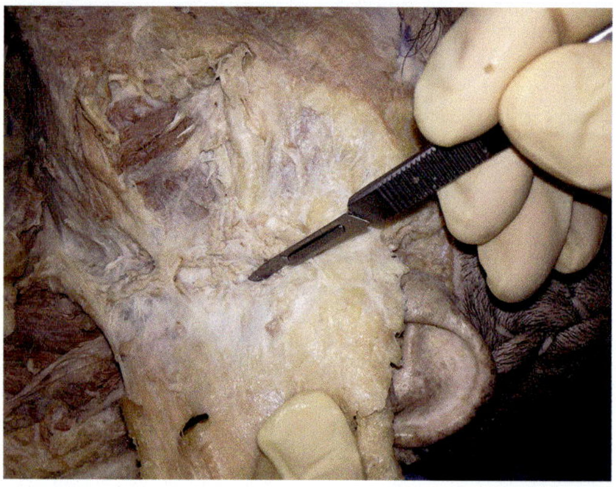

Fig. 3.96 Sharp dissection of parotid sheath over parotid duct onto the parotid gland

Clinical Correlation

Midface innervation is provided mostly by the buccal branch of the facial nerve; and innervates zygomaticus major and minor, buccinator, orbicularis oris, levator anguli oris, levator labii superioris alaeque nasi, risorius, procereus, and nasalis.

2. Identify the facial nerve branches innervating the muscles from their deep surface.

Clinical Correlation

It is important for the surgeon to remain in a plane superficial to the zygomatic major and zygomatic minor muscles to avoid injury to the facial nerve branches

3. With blunt dissection follow the buccal branch posteriorly into the parotid gland removing the parotid tissue superficial to the nerve until the buccal branch is exposed with in the gland and seen joining the other facial nerve branches to form the parotid plexus (Fig. 3.98). Ease of dissection of the parotid plexus is specimen dependent.
4. From the parotid plexus follow the other branches of the facial nerve peripherally:
   (a) The *temporal branch*, which passes in front of the tragus of the ear to pass over the zygomatic arch (Fig. 3.99).
   (b) The *zygomatic branch* between the temporal and buccal branches.

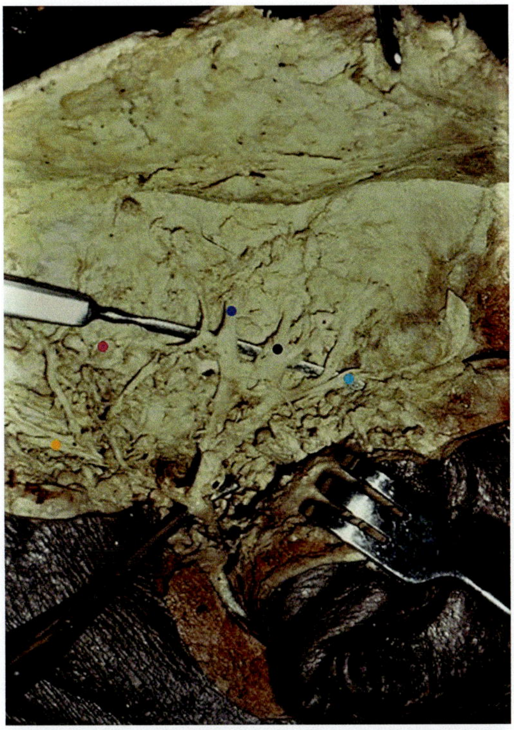

Fig. 3.98 In another specimen, the parotid plexus is exposed. Note the motor root of the facial nerve exiting in the region of the stylomastoid foramen (inferior probe), the temporal branch (teal dot), the zygomatic branch (black dot), Buccal branch (blue dot), the mandibular branch (red dot), and the cervical branch (orange dot)

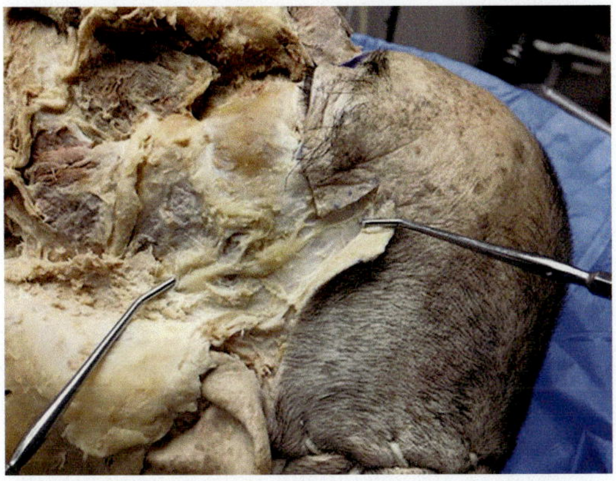

Fig. 3.99 The temporal branch of the facial nerve is shown originating from the anterior edge of the parotid (left pointer) and traveling deeply over the zygomatic arch, before it continues a more superficial course. Its temporal branches (right pointer) are seen superiorly in the superficial temporal fascia about 1.5 cm superior-lateral to the tail of the brow

Clinical Correlation

The **zygomatic branch** and the buccal branch innervate the orbicularis oculi muscle. Excision of parotid gland tumors will sacrifice facial nerve function effecting closure of the eyelids. Therefore, subsequent eyelid surgery will be necessary to reduce the risk of exposure keratopathy.

(c) The *mandibular branch* coursing parallel to the inferior margin of the mandible.

Clinical Correlation

As with much of the midface, there is extensive overlap of innervation. The risorius is supplied by both the buccal and mandibular branches of the facial nerve.

(d) The *cervical branch*, crossing the angle of the mandible to enter the neck.

5. Follow the parotid plexus branches inferiorly below the ear lobe until they combine to form the single motor root of the facial nerve. It emerges from the skull base through the stylomastoid foreman (*see* Fig. 3.98.)
6. The *posterior auricular branch* passes posterior to the ear and was dissected earlier in this dissection (Section "Ear") (*see* Fig. 3.44).

Clinical Correlations

An important anatomical concept for the facial surgeon is that the muscles of facial expression are innervated from their posterior surface, except the buccinator and levator anguli oris. Therefore, surgical midface dissection can occur in the anterior subcutaneous plane without concern for disruption of innervation to the muscles of facial expression.

Bells Palsy (facial palsy) is the sudden loss of function of the muscles of facial expression due to idiopathic injury to the seventh nerve (facial nerve). The patient will present with brow ptosis, drooping of the mouth along with inability to close the eyelids on the effected side. Trauma, vasculopathic or neoplastic processes along the course of the facial nerve also account for facial palsy. Iatrogenic injury to branches of the seventh nerve can occur during face lifting.

The Facial Artery

1. Continue the sub-SMAS dissection inferiorly to the lower border of the mandible to mobilize the jowl (Fig. 3.100).
2. At the inferior border of the mandible and at the anterior border of the masseter muscle, dissect through the platysma muscle to locate the facial artery where it crosses the mandible (Fig. 3.101). The facial artery is more tortuous and usually located anterior to the facial vein.

Clinical Correlation
At this location, the facial artery and vein are superficial and covered only by skin and platysma muscle. It is here that the facial pulse can be palpated. It is also a danger zone for injection of cosmetic facial fillers.

3. With blunt dissection, trace the facial artery superiorly toward the oral commissure and identify the inferior labial and superior labial arteries (Fig. 3.102). Note it tortuous course.
4. Continue to trace the facial artery superiorly to the lateral side of the nose where its name changes to the angular artery (Fig. 3.103).

Buccinator Muscle

This muscle is sometimes referred to as an accessory muscle of mastication due to its role in compressing the cheeks inwards against molars, thus, aiding in chewing and swallowing.

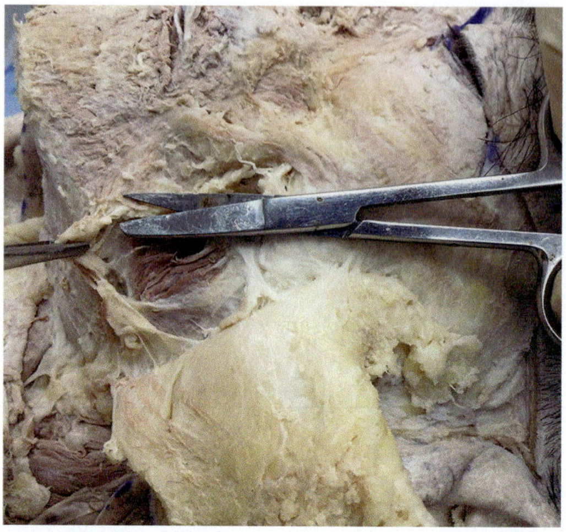

Fig. 3.100 Sub-SMAS dissection inferiorly to the lower border of the mandible

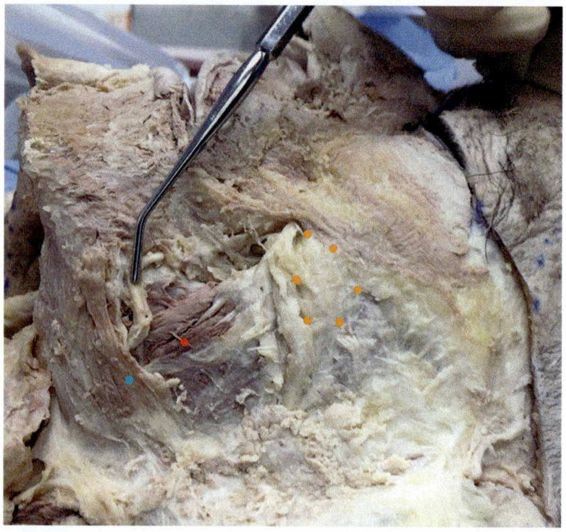

Fig. 3.101 Facial artery (pointer) where it crosses the mandible and under the lateral extension of the platysma (blue dot). Note the buccal fat pad (yellow dots), and masseter muscle (red dot)

1. Reflect the buccal fat pad medially (Fig. 3.104). It is the deep fat pad located between the buccinator muscle medially, the masseter muscle laterally.
2. Identify the underlying buccinator muscle (Fig. 3.105).
3. Identify the parotid duct piercing the buccinator muscle.
4. Note that the buccinator arises anteriorly from the outer surfaces of the alveolar pro-

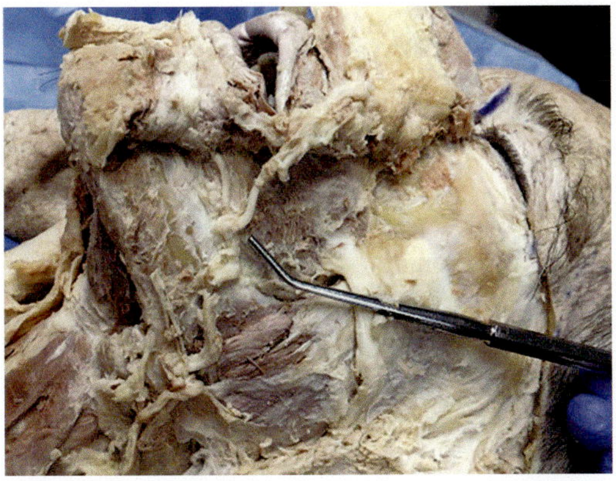

Fig. 3.102 The facial artery is seen coursing superiorly from over the angle of the mandible. The probe demonstrates its division into the superior and inferior labial arteries

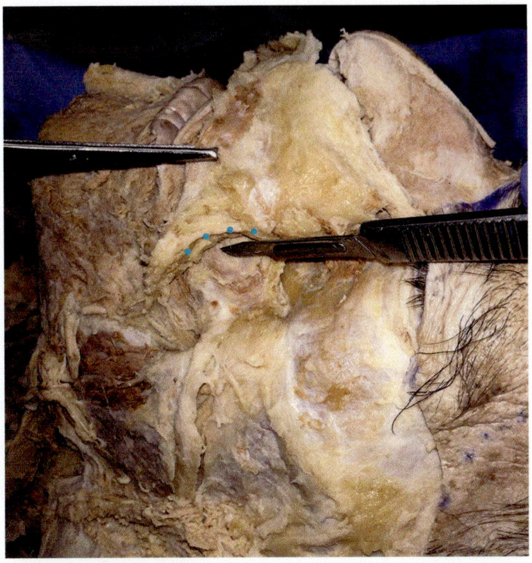

Fig. 3.104 Reflected anterior buccal fat pad (blue dots), which then extends medially

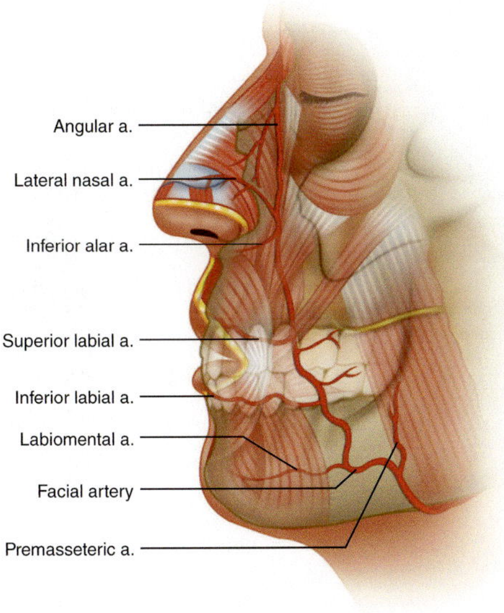

Fig. 3.103 Superior and inferior labial arteries and facial artery

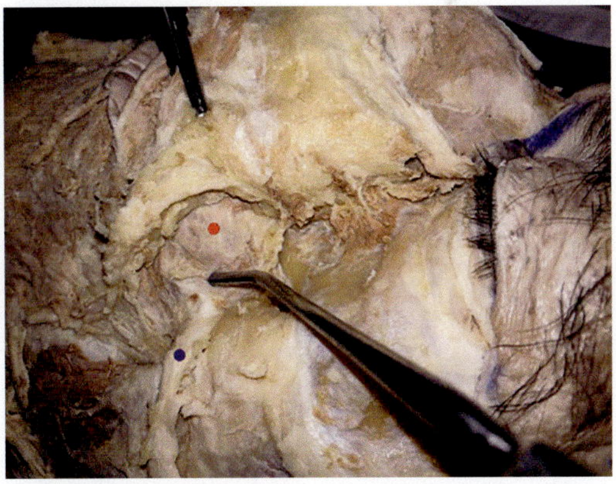

Fig. 3.105 The deep dissection has been carried medially, exposing the buccinator muscle (red dot). The probe delineates medial extension of the parotid duct (purple dot)

cesses of the maxilla and mandible, and posteriorly, from the anterior border of the pterygomandibular raphe (*see* Fig. 3.71 and 3.106).

5. Note that as the buccinator approaches the oral commissure. It fuses with the orbicularis oris muscle (Figs. 3.71 and 3.107).
6. The buccinator muscle divides into inferior and superior fibers (Fig. 3.108). Appreciate how the superior fibers travel inferiorly to become continuous with the inferior portion of the orbicularis oris. The inferior fibers become continuous with the superior orbicularis oris.
7. Coursing over the lateral surface of the buccinators muscle, identify the *long buccal nerve* which is a sensory branch of the mandibular division of the trigeminal nerve (CN V, 3rd division) (Fig. 3.109).

Clinical Correlation
It gives sensation to the gingiva near the second and third molars.

8. Recall that its motor innervation is from the buccal branch of the facial nerve (CN VII).
9. Next, with a #15 BP blade, from the anterior border of the pterygomandibular raphe carefully dissect posterior to the buccinator muscle (Fig. 3.110) until the oral cavity is entered (Fig. 3.111).
10. Note the parotid duct enters into the oral cavity through the buccinator muscle (Fig. 3.112).

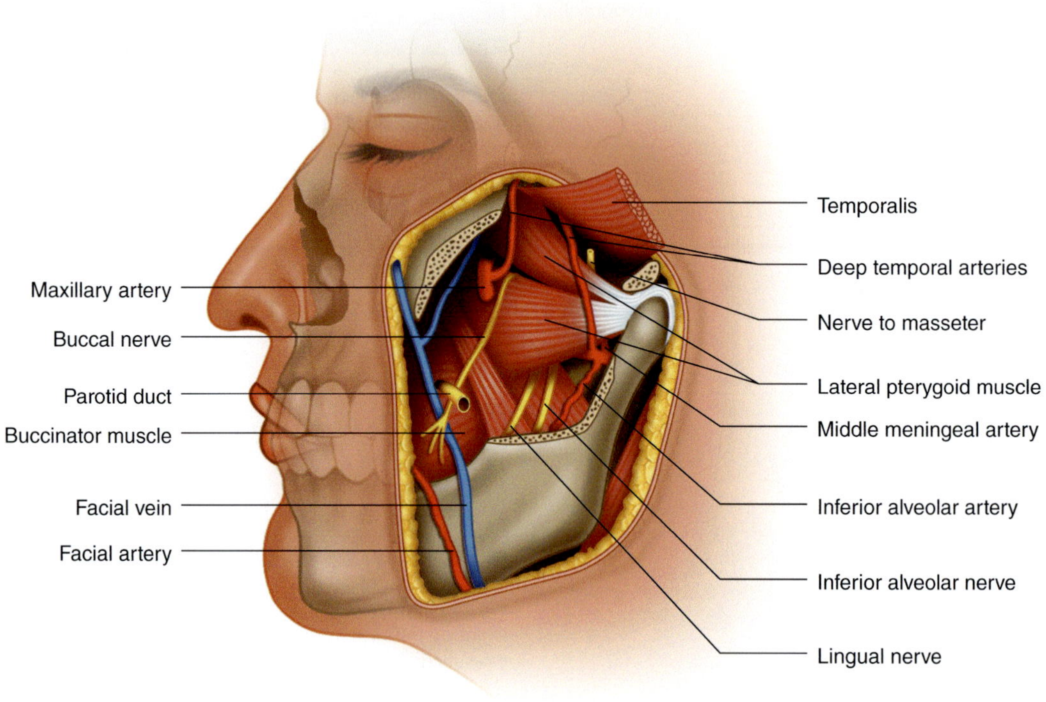

Fig. 3.106 Buccinator muscle with associated neurovascular structures

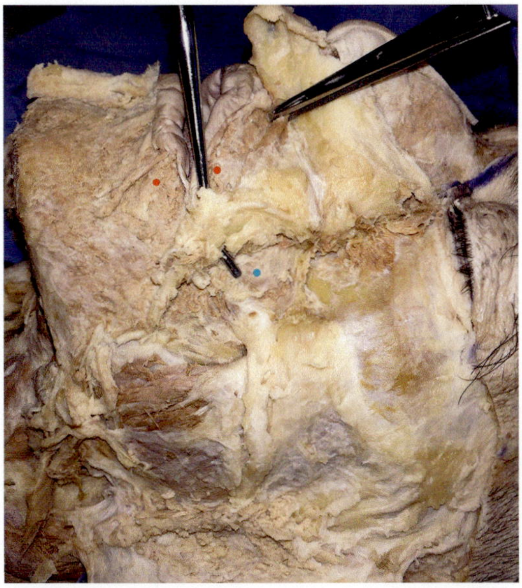

Fig. 3.107 Buccinator muscle (blue dot), demonstrating fusion with the orbicularis oris (red dots). Pointer is under reflected buccal fat)

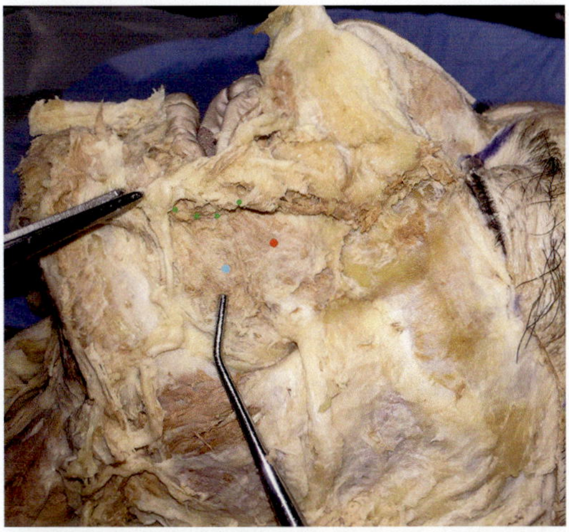

Fig. 3.108 The buccinator muscle (pointer) divides into inferior fibers (blue dot) and superior fibers (red dot). Note the orbicularis oris muscle (green dots)

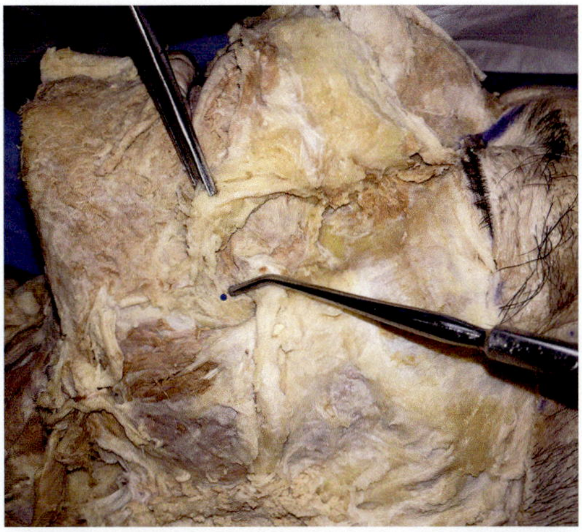

Fig. 3.109 Long buccal nerve (blue dot), which is a sensory branch of the mandibular branch of the trigeminal nerve (CN V, third division)

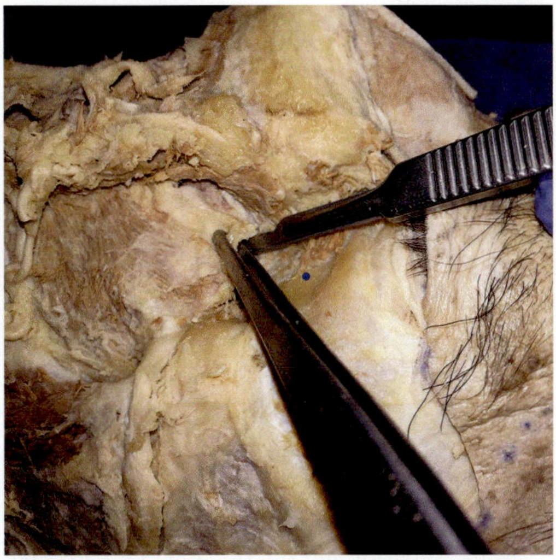

Fig. 3.110 Sub-bucinnator dissection from the pterygomandibular raphe of the maxilla (blue dot) into the oral cavity

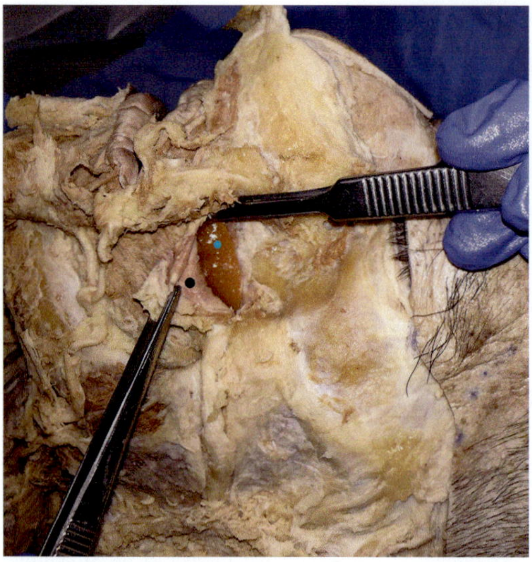

Fig. 3.111 Dissection into oral cavity. Note the reflected oral mucosa (black dot). Note the superior denture plate (blue dot) present in this cadaver

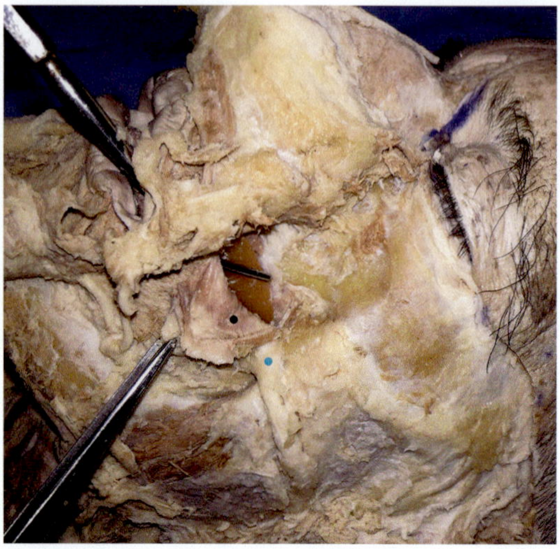

Fig. 3.112 Probe in oral cavity. Note the parotid duct (blue dot) entrance near second maxillary molar. The oral mucosa (black) is reflected in forceps

Fat Pads

The distribution of the fat pads adds to the complexity of the midface. The fat pads of the face are divided into:

1. *Subcutaneous fat* which lies above or superficial to the SMAS. As a complete unit this is generally referred to as the *malar fat pad*, and as previously discussed has four named subdivisions: nasolabial, medial, central, and lateral (*see* Fig. 3.47). In the region of the mandible, the subcutaneous fat is referred to as the superior and inferior jowl fat pads (*see* Figs. 3.55 and 3.113).
2. *Suborbicularis Oculi Fat (SOOF)* (Fig. 3.114). It is a layer of fat sandwiched beneath the orbital portion of the orbicularis oculi muscles and the periosteum of the inferior orbital rim (Fig. 3.86). Fibrous attachments may have been cut during the sub-SMAS dissection above. It is located caudal to the orbitomalar ligament. The SOOF is made up of two fat pads:
   (a) Identify the *lateral* SOOF pad which is bound superiorly by an imaginary line drawn horizontally from the lateral orbital wall. Temporally, the lateral SOOF pad abuts the deep temporal extension of the buccal fat pad. Medially, the lateral SOOF pad borders the medial SOOF fat pad.
   (b) Identify the *medial* SOOF pad as the deep fat at the inferior orbital rim. The inferior boundary of the SOOF is the tear trough. Superiorly, the medial SOOF extends over the inferior orbital rim and extends toward the tarsus.
3. *Sub-SMAS Malar Fat* (*see* Figs. 3.86 and 3.114) or the preperiosteal fat.

Identify the sub-SMAS malar fat pad, deep to the mimetic muscles. It is a large fat pad, with attachment to both the underlying zygomatic periosteum and overlying musculature.

It exhibits two components both whose superior edge abut with the inferior edge of the SOOF of the lower lid:

(a) Identify the *medial* component near the lateral border of the levator labii superioris alaeque nasi at the nasolabial fold. Trace it Inferomedially, behind the orbicularis oris into the upper lip.

Fig. 3.113 Superficial fat compartments of the cheek

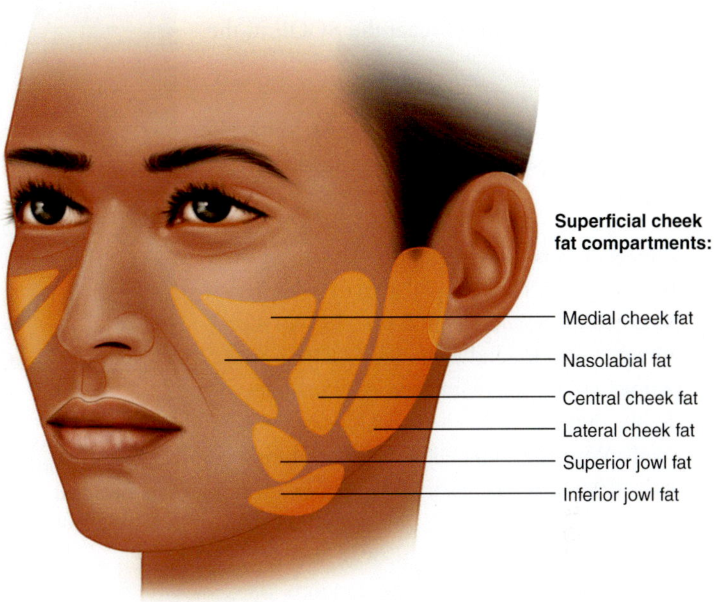

Fig. 3.114 Deep or sub-SMAS fat compartments of the eyelid and cheek

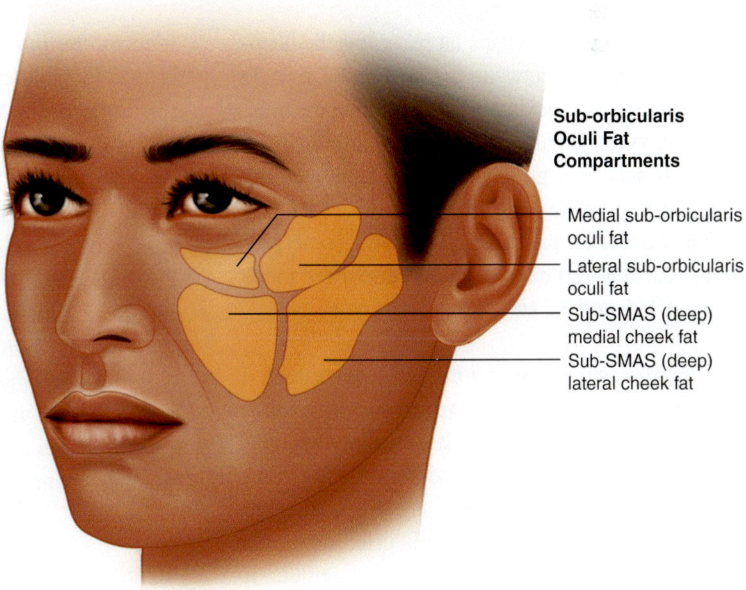

(b) Identify the *lateral* component. It is bound by the bony attachment of the SMAS to the zygoma. Superiorly it extends beyond the inferior orbital rim to meet the SOOF in the lower eyelid.

Dissect inferolaterally, to where it joins the superficial extension of the buccal fat pad.

Clinical Correlations

The sub- SMAS or deep malar fat overlies the periosteum below the orbital rim, deep to the mimetic muscles and abuts the SOOF compartment of the lower lid, providing volumetric blending across the lid- cheek junction in youth. With age, separation occurs resulting in the nasojugal and malar creases.

Retention of midface volume is key to a youthful appearance. Locations and sizes of fat pads in the subcutaneous tissue, and sub-SMAS or deep plane vary within individuals depending on a patient's age and weight.

Buccal Fat Pad

The *buccal fat pad* (Bichat's fat pad): It is the deepest fat pad located between the buccinator muscle and the more superficial muscles including the masseter, the zygomaticus major, and the zygomaticus minor. It acts as a gliding pad that facilitates the action of the muscles of mastication.

The buccal fat pad is large and sits in the preperiosteal space. It can be divided into three lobes (Figs. 3.115 and 3.116).

1. Identify the *anterior lobe*. It was reflected above (Fig. 3.104). It is triangular or rectangular in shape, overlies the oral cavity, with one vertex at the anterior edge of the buccinator, one at the levator labii superioris alaeque nasi, and one at the orbicularis oris. It extends superiorly up to the infraorbital foramen. It sits posterior to the zygomaticus major and zygomaticus minor muscles.

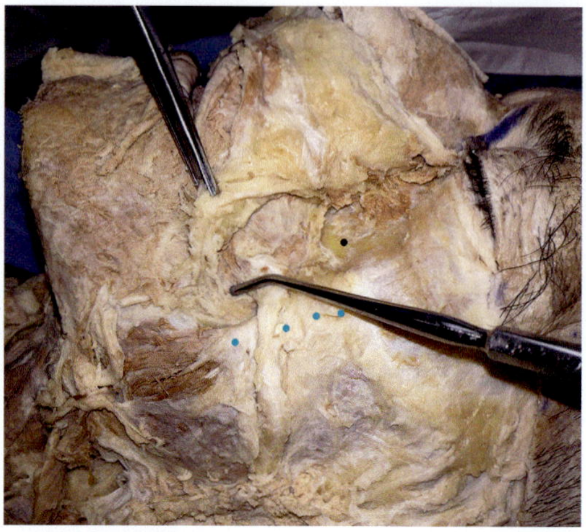

Fig. 3.115 The Buccal fat pad. The anterior lobe is reflected in forceps. The intermediate lobe is at the tip of the pointer. Portions of the posterior lobe are deep to the blue dots and not dissected in this specimen. Note the maxillary bone ((black dot)

Clinical Correlation

The parotid duct (conveying saliva to the mouth), the anterior facial vein, the infraorbital vessels, and the infraorbital nerve all pass through the anterior lobe of the buccal fat pad (Fig. 3.117).

2. Identify the *intermediate lobe* (Fig. 3.115). It is sandwiched between the anterior and posterior lobes of the buccal fat pad, overlying lateral wall of the maxilla.

Clinical Correlation

The intermediate pad is much more prominent in children and loses a significant amount of volume in adulthood from long standing chewing and sucking. Its loss of volume is implicated in the formation of hollow cheeks and nasolabial folds. It is the target of cosmetic fillers.

3. Identify the *posterior lobe*. It is a large, variable fat pad often extending from superficial to the temporalis muscle under the zygomatic

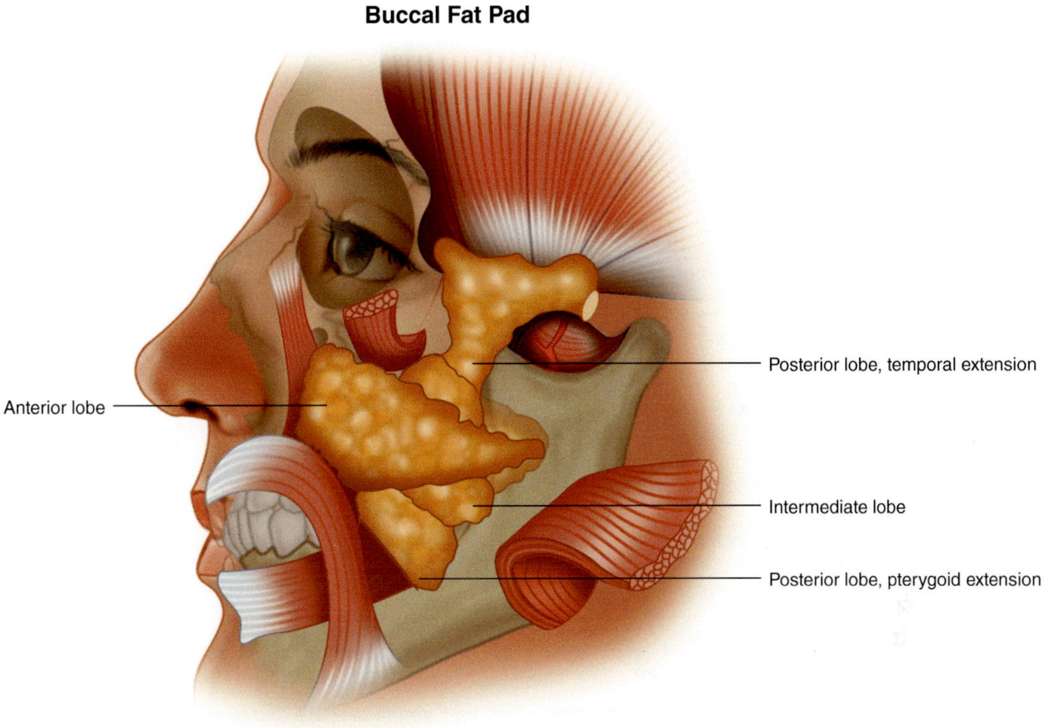

Fig. 3.116 Buccal fat pad

arch, over the inferior orbital foramen, down to the mandibular rim. Try to identify Its four segments, or processes named by location: buccal, pterygopalatine, pterygoid, and temporal processes. Some may have been sacrificed in earlier dissection.

Cadaver Dissection: Surgical Facelift

This section will review the steps of a superficial plane facelift approach and a deep plane facelift approach. This review is intended to familiarize the dissector with relevant anatomy and tissue planes (Fig. 3.118) while performing aesthetic facial surgery but is not intended to serve as a teaching tool for the steps of surgery. It is not a comprehensive surgical education manual.

Subcutaneous approach to facelifting employs a broad subcutaneous dissection to elevate and mobilize the skin for re-draping and resection to improve aesthetics. Deep plane or sub-SMAS facelifting utilizes an abbreviated subcutaneous dissection and relies on release of the facial ligaments to mobilize the SMAS along with the skin, typically in a biplanar multidirectional manner.

Superficial Facelift

Incision Design and Marking for Subcutaneous Dissection

1. When clinically marking a facelift patient, often the first point is ½ way from the superior tragus to the lateral corner of the mouth, the second point is 5–6 cm inferior to the pinna base, and the third point is midway between points 1 and 2, resulting in the dotted line as seen in (Fig. 3.119).
2. To further understand this clinical approach with cadaver dissection, extend the dissection markings anteriorly and inferiorly for anatomy demonstration purposes as follows:

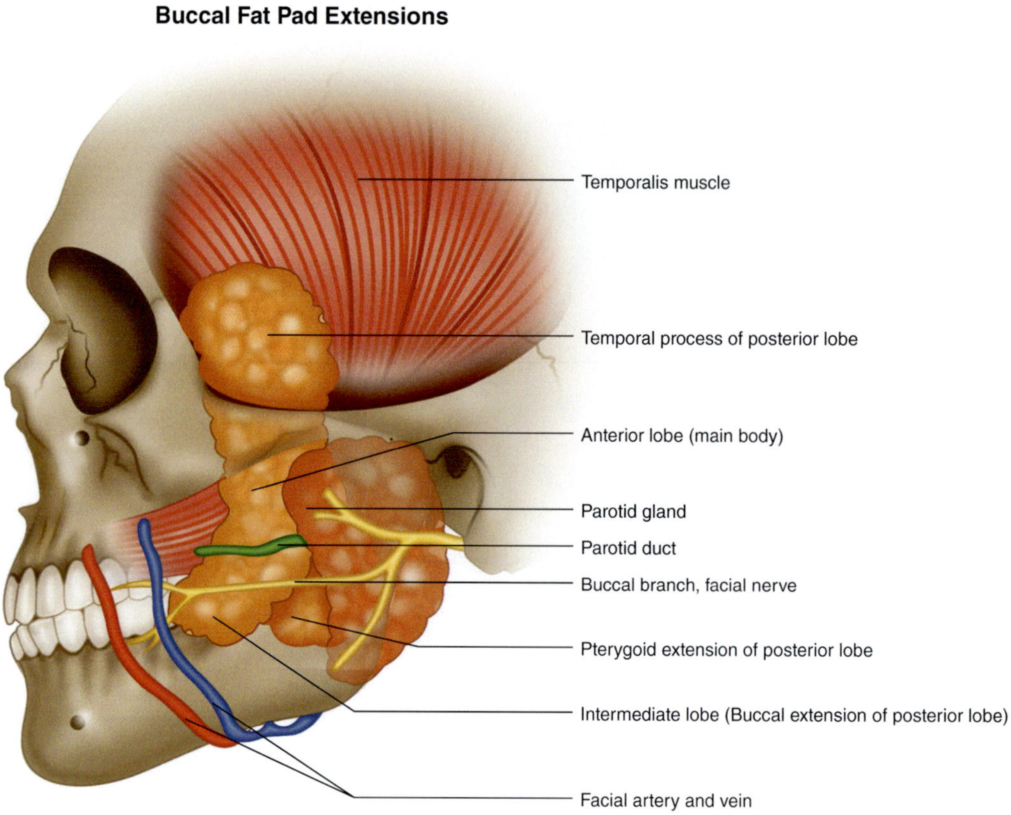

Fig. 3.117 Buccal fat pad. The parotid duct, the anterior facial vein and the buccal branch of facial nerve all pass through the anterior lobe of the buccal fat pad

Fig. 3.118 Layers of the soft tissue of the face

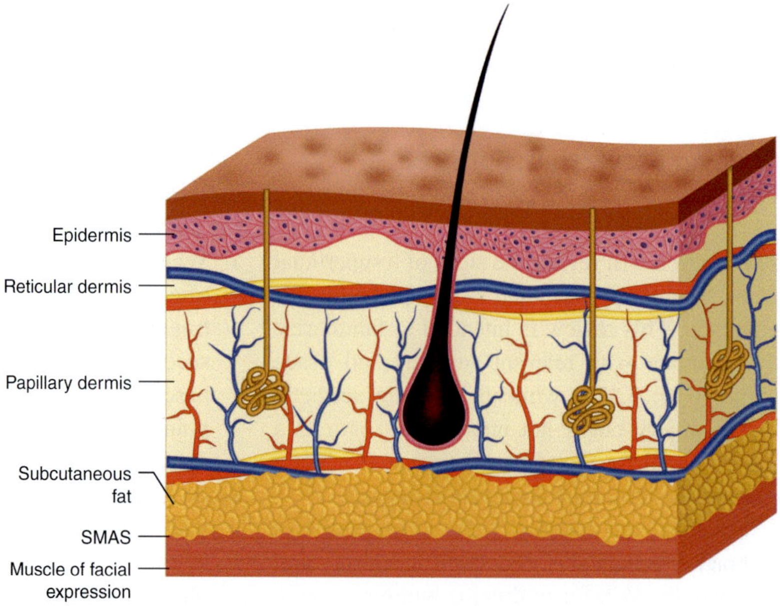

(a) First draw a mark at a point 8 cm anterior-inferiorly on an oblique line from the superior aspect of tragus to the lateral oral commissure.
(b) Second, draw a line inferiorly from the lateral palpebral canthus to the first mark.
(c) Third, draw a line to a point 9 cm inferior to the pinna base.
(d) Fourth, draw the line of incision from below the ear up along a pretragal line and extend it superoanteriorly along the anterior hairline (Fig. 3.120).

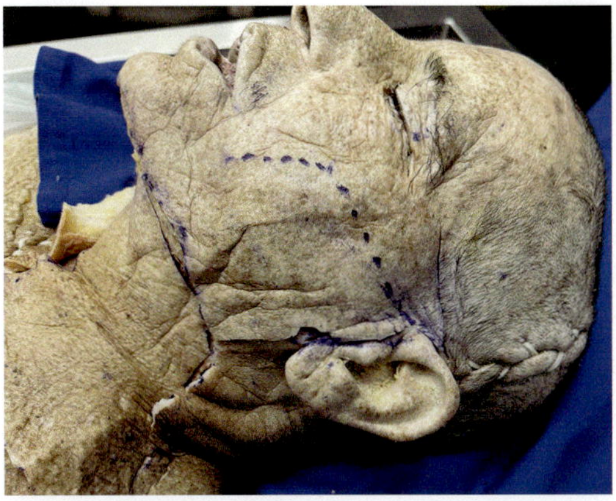

Fig. 3.119 Marking for subcutaneous dissection

Skin Layer (Subcutaneous) Elevation

1. Elevate the skin anteriorly along and within the markings. The subcutaneous attachments will be cut (Fig. 3.121).
2. Continue the elevation with a combination of blunt and sharp dissection with scissors (Figs. 3.122 and 3.123).
3. With the skin flap reflected (Fig. 3.124), the subcutaneous fat is exposed. Observe the skin thickness in the malar region thinning in the lateral periorbital region and thinning somewhat in the temporal region. It is thicker, again in the eyebrow region (see Chap. 2). It also thins in the posterior auricular region, to be dissected below.
4. As the dissection continues, note the specialized deep attachments at the orbitomalar ligament, lateral palpebral raphe and in the periorbital area.

   They were similarly encountered in Chap. 2 (Forehead and Brow, Section "Subcutaneous Dissection") to include the corrugator interdigitations at the arcus marginalis (Fig. 3.125).
5. If time allows, continue the skin elevation behind the ear (Fig. 3.126).

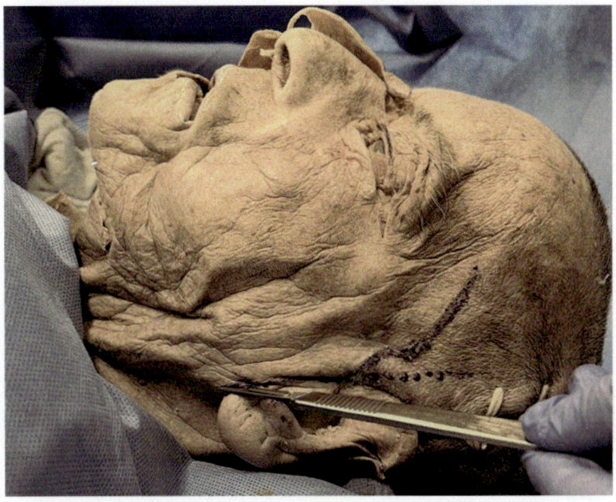

Fig. 3.120 Incision from below the pinna of the ear, passing superiorly along a pre-tragal line to continue along the hairline (solid line). The dotted line represents a superior incision alternative

Clinical Correlation

With a full incision facelift, posterior auricular extension is necessary to allow the elevated skin to be re-draped without bunching. This is continued superiorly and then camouflaged posteriorly to the hairline at the widest ear pinna width.

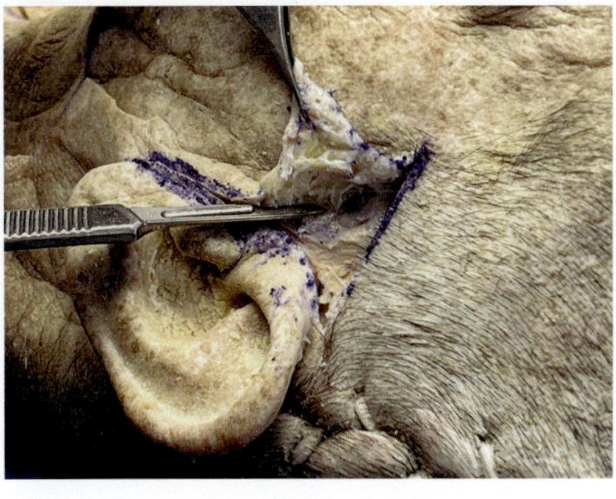

Fig. 3.121 Elevation of the skin flap starting in the malar region. Note the subcutaneous attachments

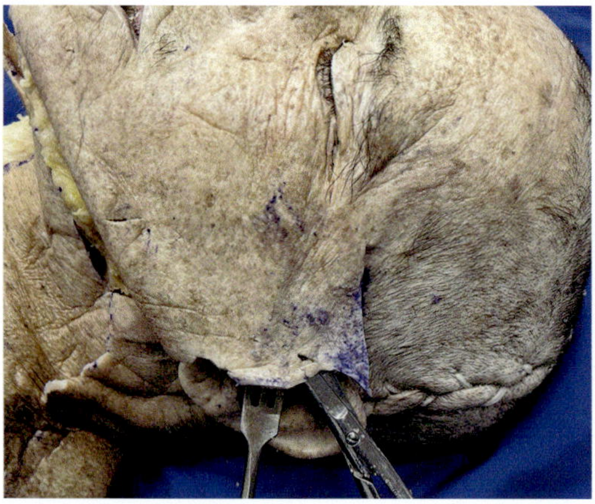

Fig. 3.122 Elevation of the skin flap with blunt and sharp dissection in the malar region

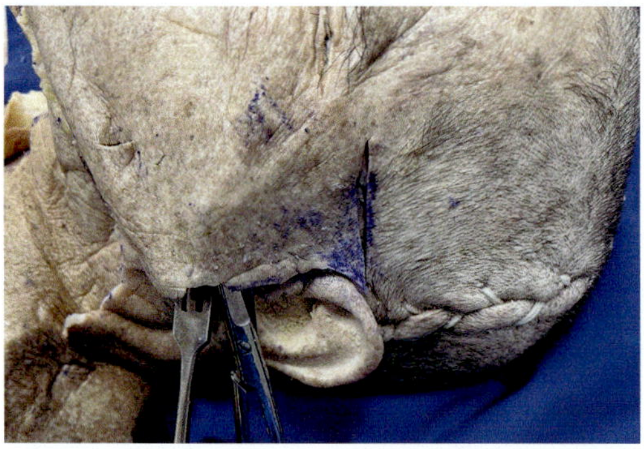

Fig. 3.123 Elevation of the skin flap inferiorly toward the angle of the mandible

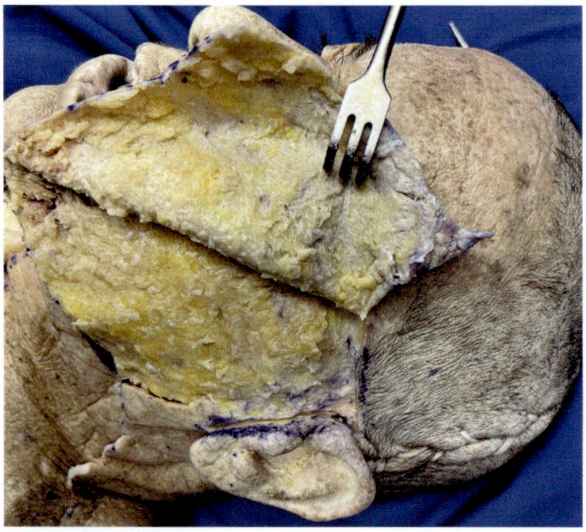

Fig. 3.124 Skin flap reflected, exposing the underlying subcutaneous fat layer

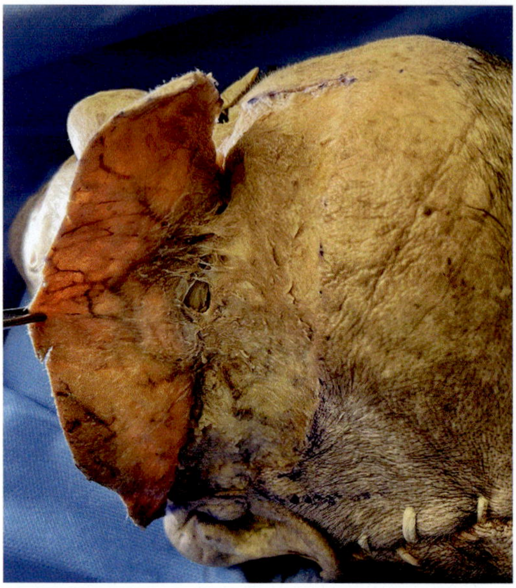

Fig. 3.125 Corrugator and orbicularis interdigitations at the superior orbital rim

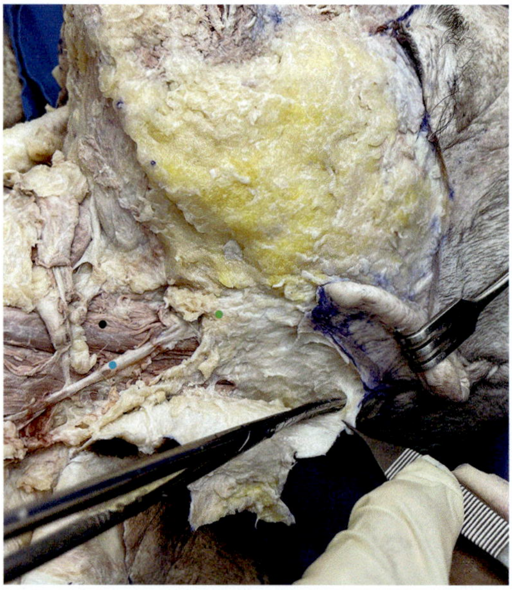

Fig. 3.126 Retro-auricular subcutaneous skin elevation. Note the greater auricular nerve within the fascia (green dot), external jugular vein (blue dot) and anterior border of Sternocleidomastoid muscle (black dot), in a deeper plane

Extreme caution must be exercised with the thin skin elevation inferior and posterior to ear to preserve the greater auricular nerve branches to the external ear. The greater auricular nerve is found at a point 6.5 cm inferior to the external auditory canal (Fig. 3.44).

SMAS Plication

1. Aesthetic facial rejuvenation is not solely reliant on skin re-draping but also relies on mobilizing the deeper facial soft tissue, namely through SMAS manipulation.
2. Once the subcutaneous dissection is complete, access is gained to the underlying SMAS layer. The SMAS is then engaged, plicated, and elevated in the desired vector, as follows:

An anchoring bite is placed, engaging the deep tissue overlying the most lateral third of the zygomatic arch. It is then used to engage the SMAS in a purse string style for distributed mobilization and lift. This can be performed with single or multiple sutures (Fig. 3.127).

Clinical Correlation
The frontal branch of the facial nerve travels along the periosteum of the zygomatic arch within the middle third, therefore the deep pass is safely placed lateral to the nerve course.

Skin Re-Draping

1. Once the SMAS is plicated, attention is then directed to skin re-draping and closure. This will be difficult in the cadaver, due to the rigid nature of the embalmed tissue.
2. The skin envelope is re-draped first around the ear. The "in-cuts" of the skin flap are made at anchoring points on the lateral zygomatic arch and the tragus.
3. Once re-draped with anchoring sutures, the surgeon determines the extent of necessary skin excision. Then closure is performed.
4. When closing the post-auricular incision, care is taken to assure optimal alignment of the hairline, to avoid an unnatural "step-off deformity."

Clinical Correlation
Natural post-operative appearance in this region relies on careful re-draping and conservative skin excision to avoid "pixie ear deformity" or an "attached earlobe." Additionally, a pre-tragal depression can be cut within the SMAS and an anchoring suture placed in the skin to this point to further the natural appearance.

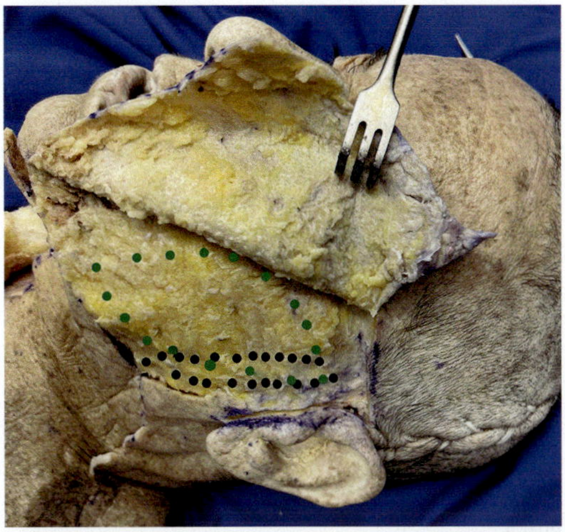

Fig. 3.127 SMAS plication with double purse string sutures. The black dots show the location of a narrow lateral purse string suture. The green dots show the location of larger central purse string suture

Deep Plane/Biplanar Facelift

Incision Design and Markings in Another Cadaver

1. Anteriorly, begin the incision sparing the temporal hair tuft (Fig. 3.128) to permit some hair removal depending on desired skin resection. Alternatively a traditional approach within the hair can be made.
2. Continue the incision inferiorly and carry over the tragus. In a male, the incision can alternatively be placed in the pre-tragal sulcus.
3. The incision is carried posteriorly around the ear lobe and over the conchal bowl, this can be continued as a pre-hairline incision which allows maximal re-draping without concern for step-off (Fig. 3.129). Alternatively, a high transverse incision can be designed into the occipital hair.
4. For concomitant neck lifting a submental incision is designed 0.5 cm behind the natural crease and is approximately 3–4 cm long (Fig. 3.130).

Surgical Steps

Neck

1. The submental incision is made with a 15 blade and blunt scissors used to develop a subcutaneous plane (Fig. 3.131).
2. A retractor is introduced to facilitate view into the deeper pocket. To carry the dissection laterally, holes can be poked within the fat. The planes of dissection are connected with facelift scissors to cut into and connect the channels. The inferior extent of the dissection is typically to the thyroid cartilage.
3. Notice the subcutaneous, and pre-platysmal fat (Fig. 3.132).

Clinical Correlation

It is the pre-platysmal fat, *not* the subcutaneous fat, that is the target for submental liposuction.

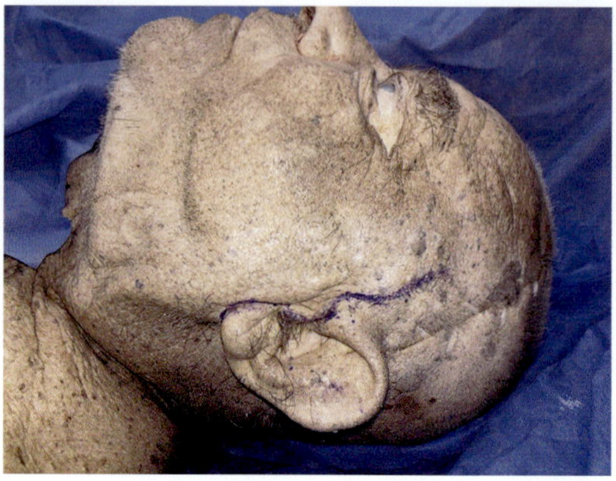

Fig. 3.128 The planned anterior aspect of the deep plane face lift incision is shown; a course anterior to the temporal hair tuft and around the tragus is shown

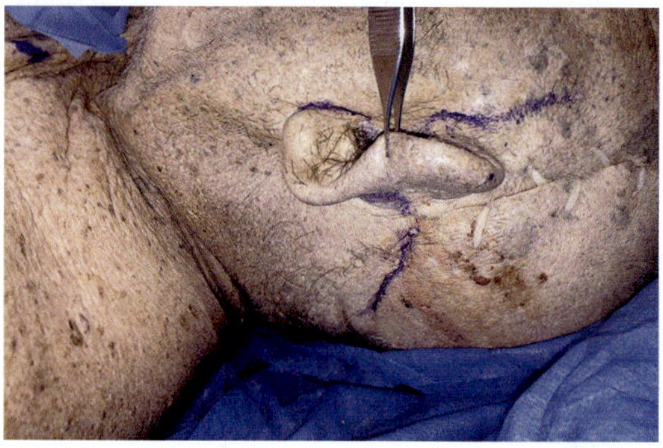

Fig. 3.129 The planned posterior course of the facelift incision is shown extending around the ear lobe, over the conchal bowl and continuing in this example along the inferior aspect of the hairline

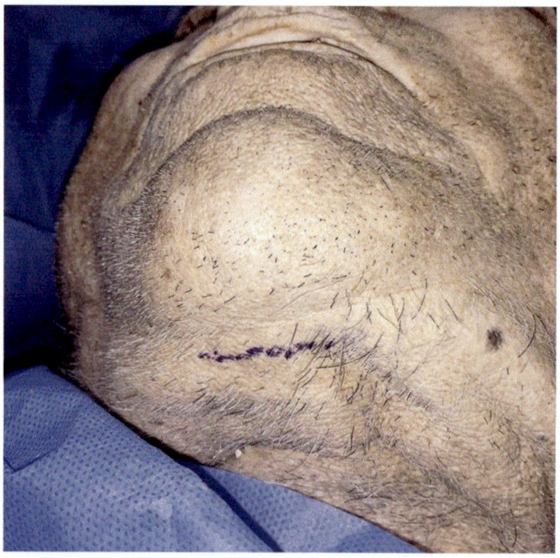

Fig. 3.130 The planned submental incision is shown, designed 1 cm posterior to the submental crease and 3–4 cm in length

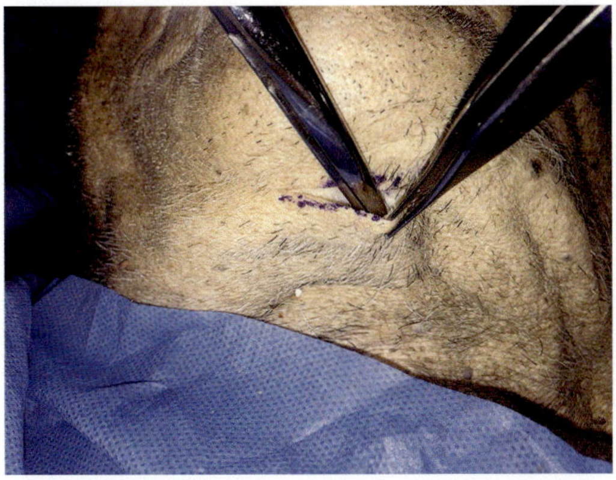

Fig. 3.131 Blunt scissors are being used to perform the subcutaneous dissection within the submental incision. This is continued inferiorly and laterally

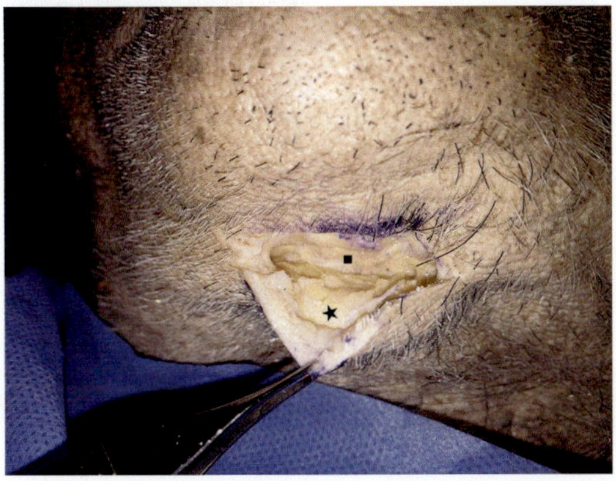

Fig. 3.132 The skin flap of the neck dissection is reflected to demonstrate the subcutaneous fat (star) and pre-platysmal fat (square)

4. Next, mark a "point of safety," 4 cm from the angle of the mandible (Fig. 3.133). Be aware that the marginal mandibular nerve branch crosses the facial artery about 3 cm anterior to the mandibular angle.

Clinical Correlation

The posterior 4 cm of the mandible is considered a danger zone.[1]

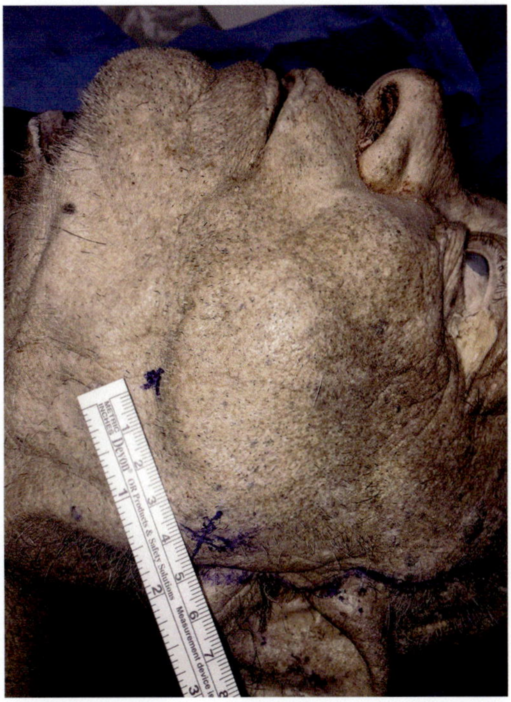

Fig. 3.133 A ruler is used to demonstrate the danger zone where the marginal mandibular nerve branch often travels superficially over the facial artery and is vulnerable to injury. This was found on average to be about 3 cm anterior to the gonion (X ink mark). The danger zone is therefore prudently marked at 4 cm (blue ink dot)

Surgical dissection along the mandible is performed in a subcutaneous plane to the "point of safety" to avoid injury to the marginal mandibular branch. Injury to the marginal mandibular nerve compromises the depressor angulii oris muscle.

5. Through the submental incision, continue the subcutaneous dissection laterally to the "point of safety," as marked above in step 4 (Fig. 3.134).
6. Once the platysmal edge is visualized, resect the platysma using an elliptical style incision with pre-planned dog ears inferiorly to avoid redundancy (Fig. 3.135).

Clinical Correlation
This facilitates advancement in the horizontal plane which helps create the cervicomental angle and reduces banding.

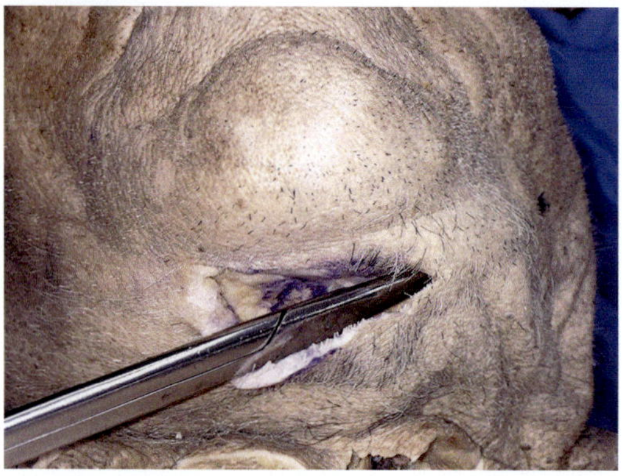

Fig. 3.134 Lateral subcutaneous dissection through the submental incision is shown, care taken to avoid continuing laterally beyond the point of safety (blue ink dot) toward the marginal mandibular nerve

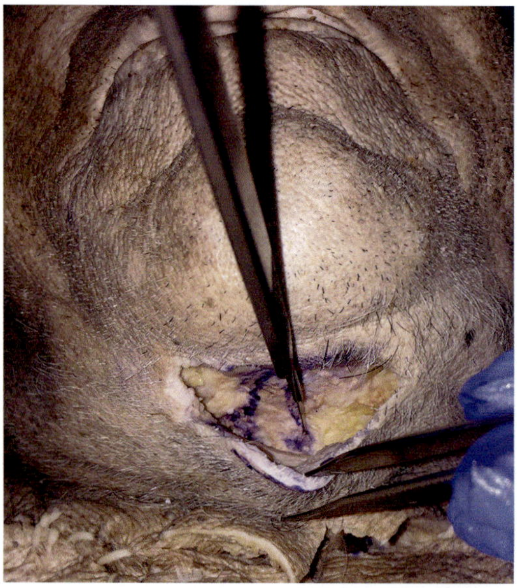

Fig. 3.135 Once dissection is complete and the platysma is identified an elliptical style incision can be made with pre-placed inferior "dog ears." A scalpel is used to incise the marked incision within the platysma

7. 3–0 Mersilene or monocryl is used to engage the pre-hyoid tissue and the cut platysmal edges. Multiple horizontal sutures are placed as the closure is continued superiorly toward the chin. For demonstration purposes this is shown with a silk suture as the platysmal edges are drawn together (Fig. 3.136).
8. The submandibular gland may be encountered, and if enlarged, it can be manipulated for optimal cosmetic rejuvenation.

Clinical Correlation
The facial artery and vein run obliquely over the posterior portion of the gland, and the marginal mandibular nerve can run across the superior aspect of the gland. The lingual nerves and hypoglossal run superiorly and inferiorly to the deep process of the gland respectively. All these critical structures are extracapsular, so if manipulation is undertaken, intracapsular gland manipulation permits a safer approach.

9. Next, the submental incision is meticulously closed.

Face

1. Use a 15 or 10 blade to initiate the facelift incision (Fig. 3.137). The initial 2 cm flap elevation is preferably performed with a 10 blade because the skin is densely adherent to the pre-auricular fascia with little intervening subcutaneous fat (Fig. 3.138).
2. Next the facelift scissors can be used to continue the subcutaneous dissection anteriorly 2–4 cm beyond the marked line of deep plane entry (Fig. 3.139).
   (a) The deep plane entry point extends from the gonion to the lateral canthus. This places the area of SMAS manipulation anterior to the lateral more adherent SMAS for fixation.
3. The dissection is carried below the mandible so the lateral platysma can be accessed (Fig. 3.140). This is performed using facelift scissors to create channels for advance-

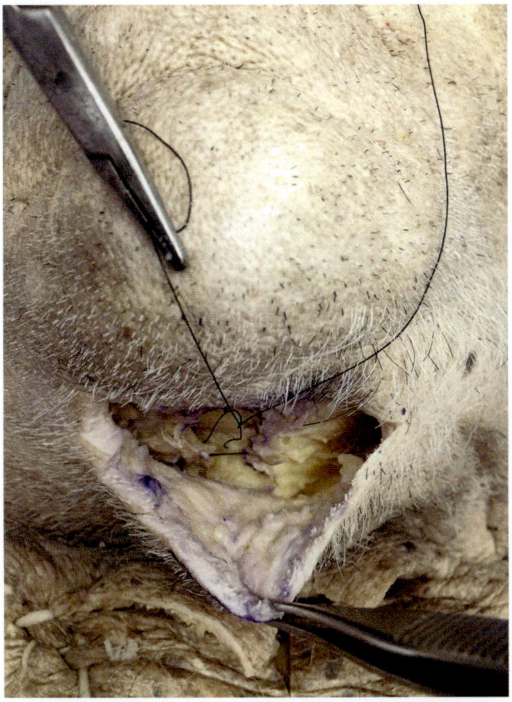

Fig. 3.136 After platysmal resection, the pre-hyoid tissue is engaged followed by each platsymal edge and the suture is tied to horizontally tighten the platysma and improve the aesthetics of the cervicomental angle

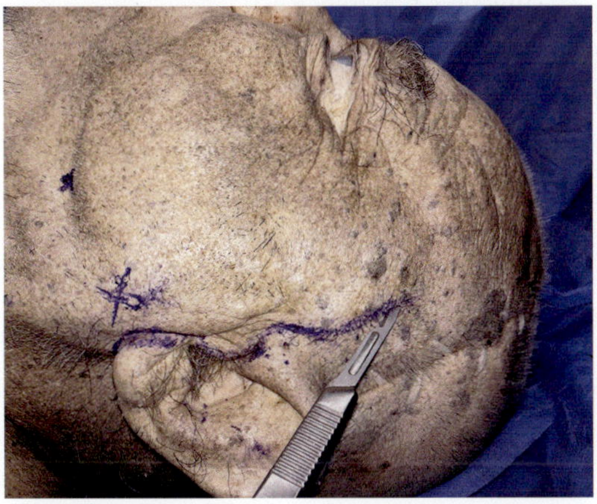

Fig. 3.137 The blade is used to incise the previously marked facelift incision

ment which are then carefully sharply connected.

4. Inferiorly beyond the mandible and posteriorly, the flap is raised. Care should be taken to look for the fascia of the sternocleidomastoid muscle (SCM). The posterior auricular nerve will run along the anterior border of the muscle (McKinney's point 6.5 cm inferior to the external auditory canal) (Fig. 3.126).
5. Make an incision in the SMAS along the length of the pre-tragal skin incision. Preserve a 1 cm cuff for suture fixation (Fig. 3.141).
6. Dissection can be sharp until the anterior border of the partoid where the transition is

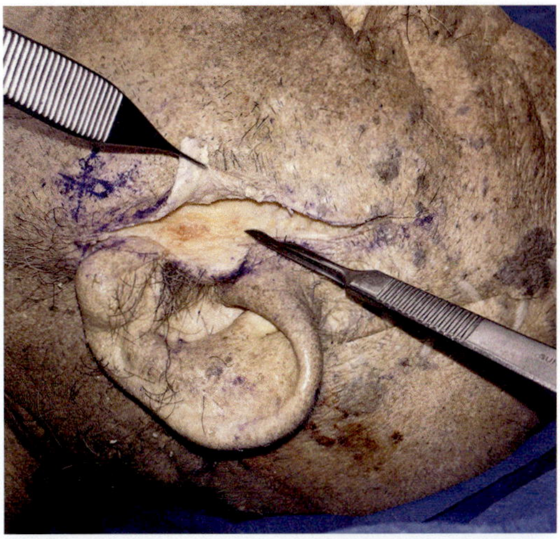

Fig. 3.138 Initial subcutaneous dissection is performed with a blade due to adherence to the underlying plane

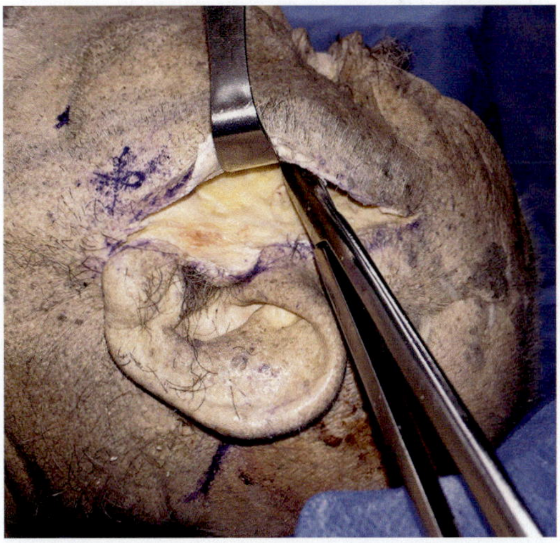

Fig. 3.139 After the initial sharp dissection the blunt scissors are used to continue the dissection anteriorly

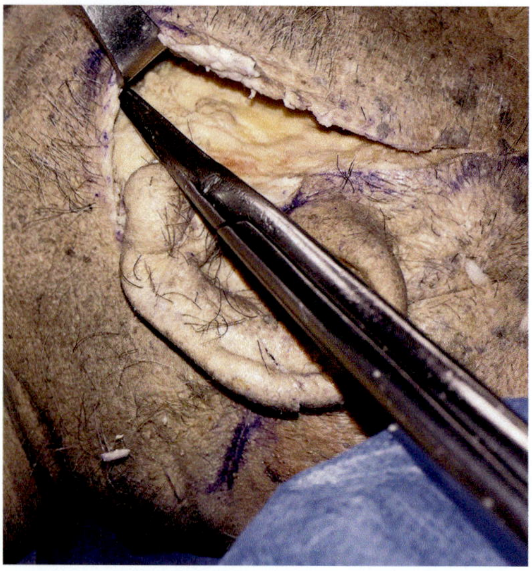

Fig. 3.140 The dissection is carried inferiorly beyond the mandible, toward the neck dissection to access the platysma

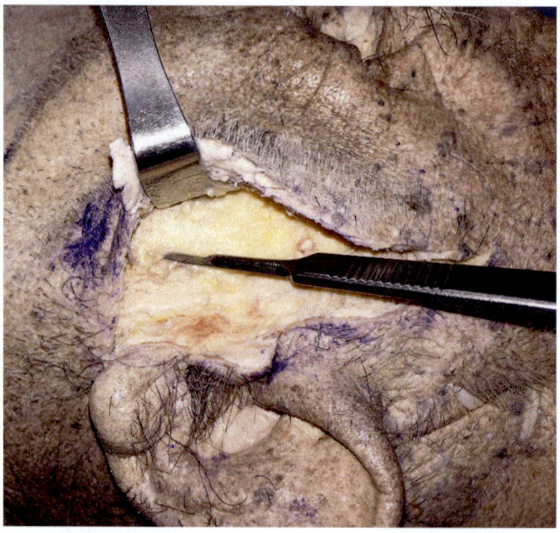

Fig. 3.141 The deep plane entry point is designed as a continuous line from the angle of the mandible superiorly to the level of the lateral canthus. The entry is being initiated here with a scalpel

made to blunt dissection, as the facial nerve branches will be exiting the anterior border of the partoid.

7. Ligamentous release is then performed to facilitate SMAS mobilization, namely the malar and masseteric cutaneous ligaments are released using vertical spreading (Fig. 3.142).

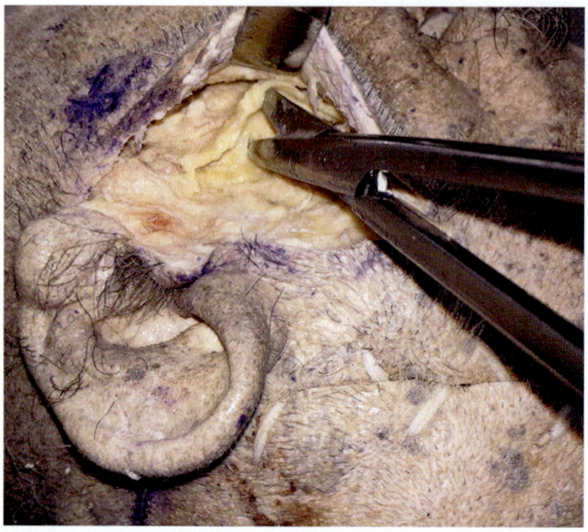

Fig. 3.142 Once the flap is raised, blunt dissection with vertical spreading is employed to avoid nerve injury. This technique is utilized to release the malar and masseteric cutaneous ligaments

8. The extent of SMAS undermining is to gain access to the ligamentous release which lie just anterior to the zygomaticus major muscle and anterior to the parotid.
9. Once adequate release is achieved the SMAS is elevated and secured, SMAS resection or plication can be performed depending on the surgeon's preference.
10. The SMAS is secured to the deep fascia, with the surgeon's suture of choice. Due to cadaver rigidity, tissue advancement is not shown, but a silk suture is used to demonstrate deep fascia and SMAS engagement (Fig. 3.143). Interrupted mattress or running locking sutures can be used along its length to the base of the ear. Posteriorly, the SMAS is similarly secured. Lastly, the skin is re-draped (Fig. 3.144). This is first performed around the ear. It is secured to the previously formed pre-tragal depression.

Clinical Correlation

To avoid pixie ear deformity, the first incision for re-draping the skin is continued along the base of the ear to the point of the lobule. The lobule is secured to the skin and deeper tissue. The skin is re-draped and resected as needed and the incision is closed.

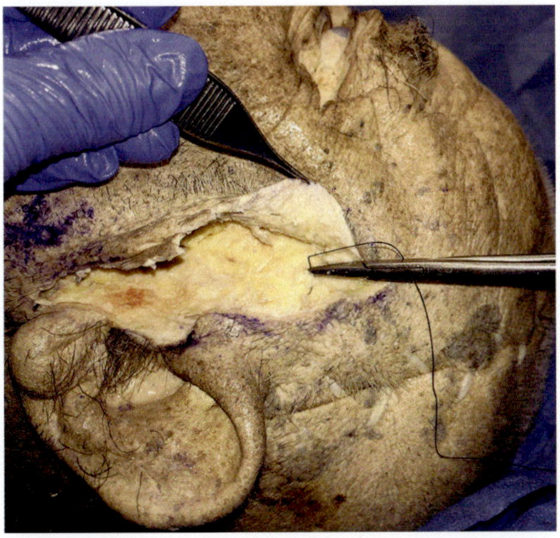

Fig. 3.143 Once release is achieved the SMAS flap will be elevated and secured to the deep fascia and posterior anterior SMAS, a pre-placed suture is shown engaging the deep fascia, prior to SMAS engagement

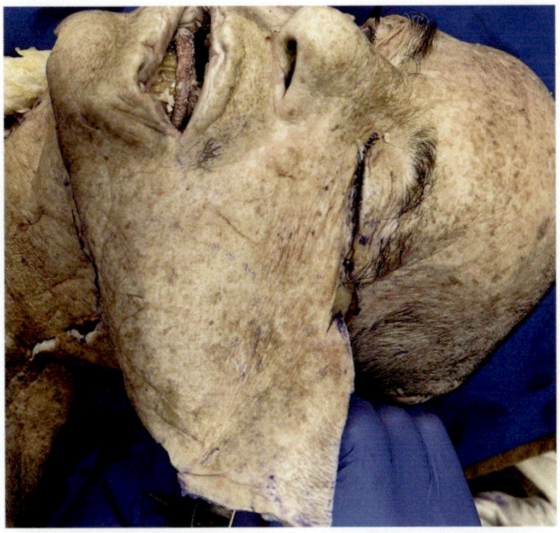

Fig. 3.144 Mobilization and re-draping of skin before in-cuts at tragus and lobule

Further Reading

Bedrossian EH, Schmidt RS, Della Rocca RC, Lemke BN. Anatomy of the eyelid, orbit, and lacrimal system: a dissection manual. Cham: Springer; 2022.

Brandy D. The QuickLift: featuring an encircling double purse-string plication technique with blunt neck/jowl undermining and small submental Tuck for tightening the sagging superficial musculoaponeurotic system, platysma, and skin. Am J Cosmet Surg. 2005;22:22.223-232.

Brennan PA, Mahadevan V, Evans BT. Clinical head and neck anatomy for surgeons. Boca Raton, FL: CRC Press, Taylor & Francis Group; 2016.

Gierloff M, Stöhring C, Buder T, Gassling V, Açil Y, Wiltfang J. Aging changes of the midfacial fat compartments: a computed tomographic study. Plast Reconstr Surg. 2012;129:263–73.

Hazani R, Chowdhry S, Mowlavi A, Wilhelmi BJ. Bony anatomic landmarks to avoid injury to the marginal mandibular nerve. Aesthet Surg J. 2011;31(3):286–9.

Hiatt JL, Gartner LP. Textbook of head and neck anatomy. 4th ed. Philadelphia, PA: Lippincott Williams & Wilkins; 2010.

Jacono A, Bryant LM. Extended deep plane facelift: incorporating facial retaining ligament release and composite flap shifts to maximize midface, jawline and neck rejuvenation. Clin Plastic Surg. 2018;45:527–54.

Moore KL, Dalley AF, Agur AMR. Clinically oriented anatomy. 7th ed. Philadelphia, PA: Lippincott Williams & Wilkins; 2014.

Netter F. Atlas of human anatomy. 7th ed. Philadelphia, PA: Saunders; 2019.

Niamtu JDMD III. FAACS cosmetic facial surgery. 3rd ed. Amsterdam: Elsevier; 2022.

Owsley JQ, Roberts CL. Some anatomical observations on midface aging and long-term results of surgical treatment. Plast Reconstr Surg. 2008;121(1):258–68.

Ozturk CN, Larson JD, Ozturk C, Zins JE. The SMAS and fat compartments of the nose: an anatomical study. Aesth Plast Surg. 2013;37(1):11–5.

Palastanga N, Soames R. Anatomy and human movement: structure and function. 6th ed. Edinburgh: Churchill Livingstone; 2012.

Standring S. Gray's Anatomy. 41st ed. Edinburgh: Elsevier Churchill Livingstone; 2016.

Zhang HM, Yan YP, Qi KM, Wang JQ, Liu ZF. Anatomical structure of the buccal fat pad and its clinical adaptations. Plast Reconstr Surg. 2002;109(7):2509–18.

The Neck

4

Richard R. Schmidt, Edward H. Bedrossian Jr., Bradley N. Lemke, and Alison H. Watson

The anatomy of the neck is complex as it represents a transition zone between the head and the thorax. Within the neck region there are many important structures including major vessels of the cardiovascular system (carotid arteries, vertebral arteries, and jugular veins), spinal cord, various peripheral nerves, portions of the gastrointestinal system (pharynx and esophagus), respiratory system (larynx and trachea), and finally the endocrine system (thyroid and parathyroid glands).

In this chapter, the study of neck anatomy is divided into superficial and deep dissections. For the purpose of the ophthalmologist, oculofacial plastic surgeon, cosmetic facial plastic surgeon, and dermatologist, this chapter will focus primarily on the superficial dissections. Although we will address more deeply placed structures out of caution, there are other excellent dissection manuals for head and neck surgeons interested in the deeper dissections of the neck.

First, the surface landmarks, cross-sectional anatomy, and triangles of the neck will be reviewed. Next the skin with be reflected. Then the underlying subcutaneous fat and platysma muscle will be reflected. The boundaries of the posterior and anterior triangles will be identified. The external jugular vein, and several cutaneous branches of the cervical plexus (posterior auricular nerve, and transverse cervical) will be dissected.

Richard R. Schmidt has died before the publication of this book.

R. R. Schmidt, PhD (Deceased)
Department of Pathology, Anatomy and Cell Biology, Sydney Kimmel Medical College of Thomas Jefferson University, Philadelphia, PA, USA

E. H. Bedrossian Jr., MD, FACS (✉)
Wills Eye Hospital, Sydney Kimmel Medical College of Thomas Jefferson University, Philadelphia, PA, USA

Department of Oculoplastic and Orbital Surgery, Wills Eye Hospital, Philadelphia, PA, USA

Clinical Professor Ophthalmology, Lewis Katz School of Medicine at Temple University, Philadelphia, PA, USA

B. N. Lemke, MD, FACS
Lemke Facial Surgery, Madison, WI, USA

Department of Ophthalmology and Visual Sciences, School of Medicine and Public Health, University of Wisconsin-Madison, Madison, WI, USA
e-mail: lemke@lemkefacialsurgery.com

A. H. Watson, MD, FACS
Department of Oculoplastic and Orbital Surgery, Wills Eye Hospital, Philadelphia, PA, USA
e-mail: awatson@willseye.org

E. H. Bedrossian Jr et al. (eds.), *Anatomy of the Forehead, Face, and Neck*,
https://doi.org/10.1007/978-3-031-56140-5_4

Surface and Cross-Sectional Anatomy of the Neck

1. Review the surface anatomy including the inferior border of the *mandible*, the *clavicle*, the *suprasternal notch*, *sternocleidomastoid muscle* (*including its sternal and clavicular attachments and the laryngeal prominence*) (Fig. 4.1).
2. Study the cross-sectional anatomy of the neck at the level of C-7 (Fig. 4.2).
   (a) Posteriorly, note the *cervical vertebral column* and the muscles that move it, e.g., trapezius, and more deeply situated vertebral muscles.
   (b) Anteriorly, and important for the following dissection, note the *platysma muscle*, *superficial and deep cervical fascia*, *thyroid and parathyroid glands, and sternocleidomastoid* muscle.

In Fig. 4.2, note the following:

- Investing layer of deep cervical fascia.
- Pretracheal fascia.
- Prevertebral fascia.
- Carotid sheath containing carotid artery, internal jugular vein, and vagus nerve.
- Cervical vertebra.
- Trapezius and sternocleidomastoid muscles.
- Thyroid gland.
- Sternohyoid, sternothyroid, and omohyoid muscles.

Fig. 4.1 Surface landmarks of the neck

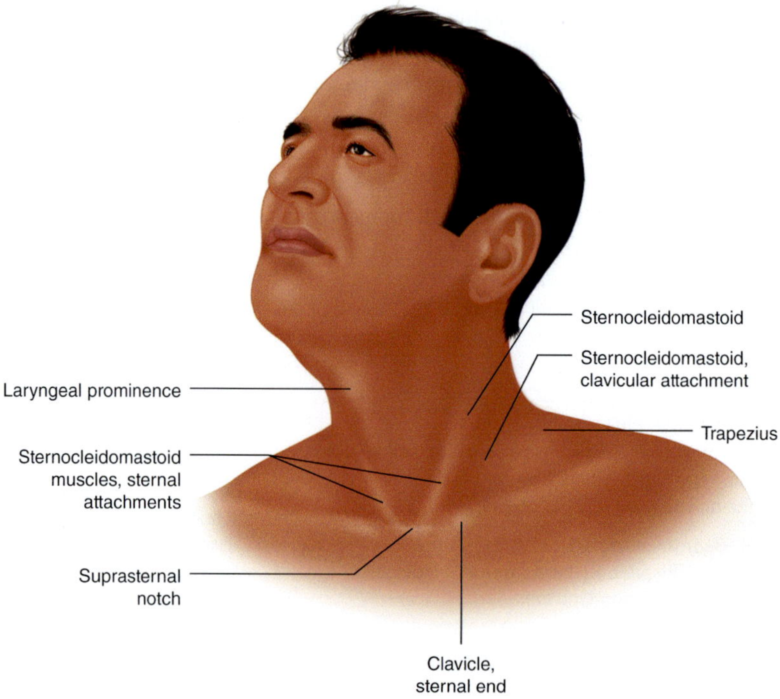

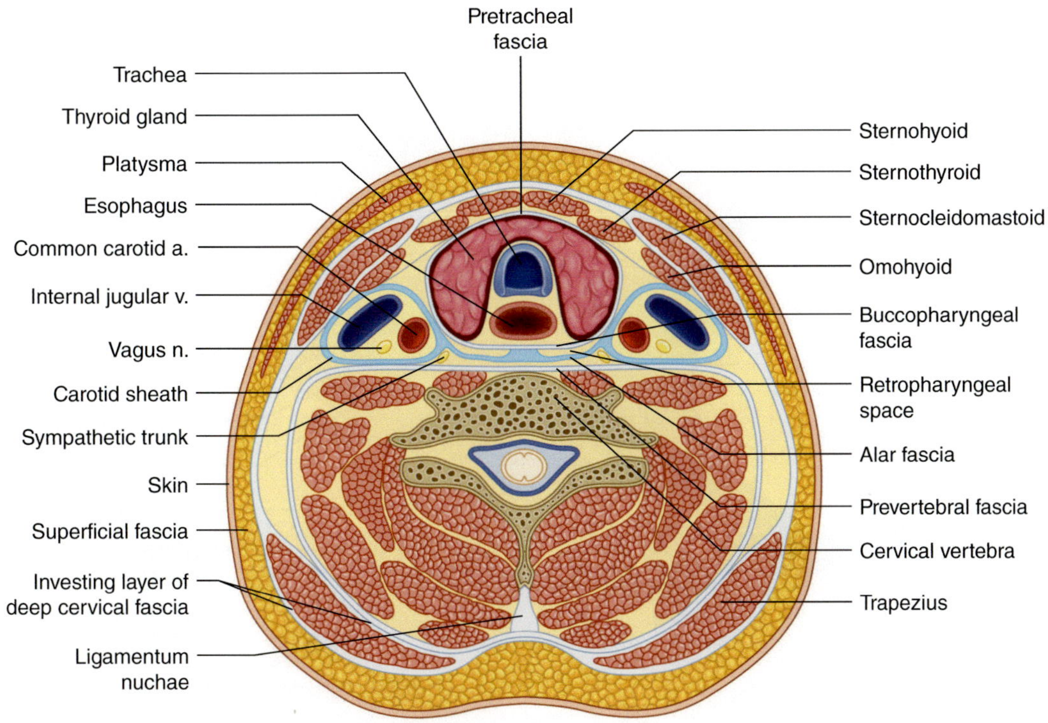

Fig. 4.2 Cross-section anatomy of the neck at the level of CV7

Triangles of the Neck

The neck is divided into a posterior triangle and an anterior by the obliquely positioned sternocleidomastoid muscle. For descriptive purposes, review their boundaries.

Posterior Triangle of the neck boundaries (Figs. 4.3, 4.4, and 4.5):

Anterior: The posterior border of the sternocleidomastoid muscle.

Posterior: the anterior border of the trapezius muscle.

Inferior: the middle one-third of the clavicle.

Superficial (*roof*)*:* investing layer of the deep cervical fascia.

Deep (*floor*)*:* deep lateral neck muscles (scalene muscles covered by prevertebral fascia).

The posterior triangle is further divided inferiorly into a smaller **subclavian** (supraclavicular) **triangle** and superiorly a much larger **occipital triangle** delineated by the inferior belly of the Omohyoid muscle. Note that the occipital triangle is divided by the accessory nerve (CN XI) into equal upper and lower portions (Fig. 4.3).

> **Clinical Correlation**
> The upper portion of the occipital triangle contains few structures of clinical significance, whereas the lower portion contains numerous significant structures. When operating in the occipital triangle, the neck surgeon must take extra care when dissection is inferior to the accessory nerve than when dissection is superior to the nerve (Figs. 4.4 and 4.5).

Anterior Triangle of the neck boundaries:

Medial: *median plane of the neck.*

Lateral: The anterior border of the *sternocleidomastoid muscle.*

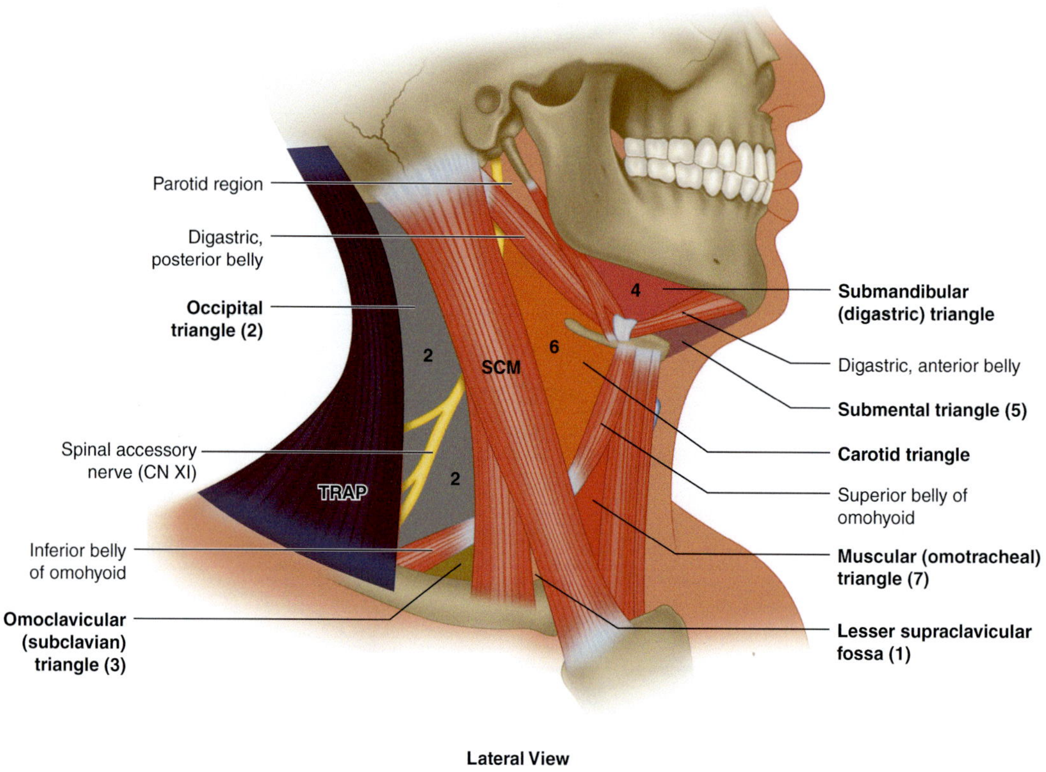

Fig. 4.3 Triangles of the neck

Superior: inferior border of the *mandible.*

Superficial (roof): investing layer of the deep cervical fascia.

Deep (floor): Contents of muscular and carotid triangles; submandibular triangle; larynx and pharynx.

The anterior triangle is further divided by the digastric and superior belly of the omohyoid muscles into smaller triangles: **muscular, carotid, submandibular,** and **submental.** The posterior belly of the digastric (and stylohyoid) separates the carotid triangle from the submandibular triangle (Fig. 4.3); the superior belly of the Omohyoid separates the carotid triangle from the muscular triangle (Figs. 4.3 and 4.6). The region between paired anterior bellies of the Digastric muscles and the body of the hyoid bone is the unpaired submental triangle (Fig. 4.7).

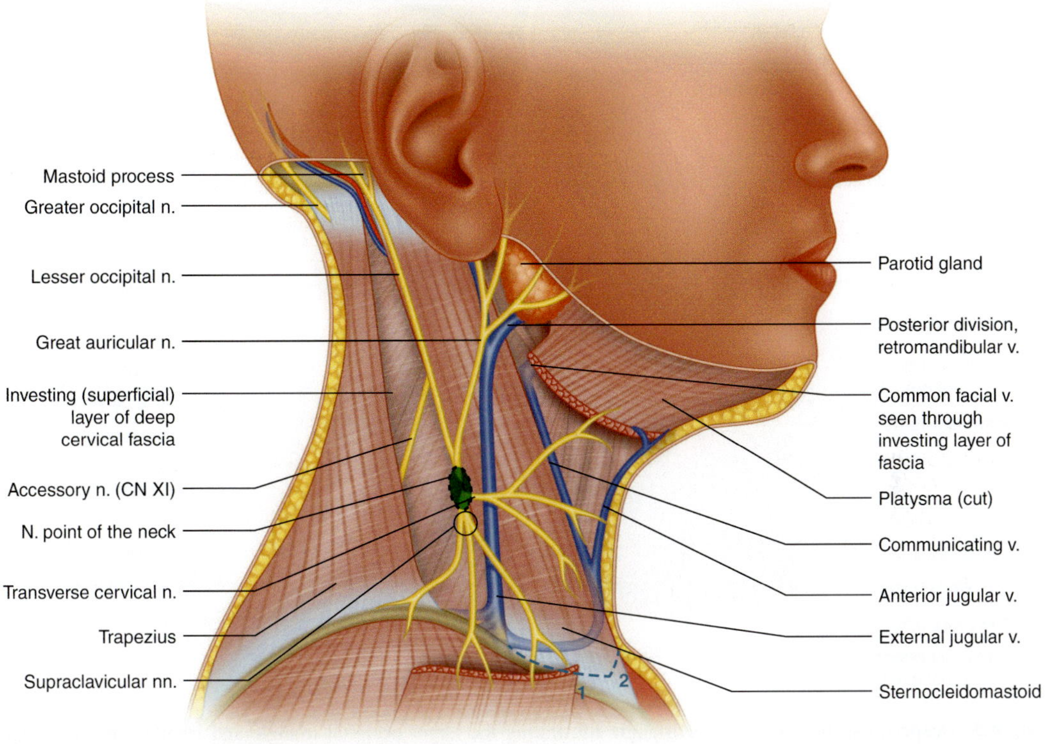

Fig. 4.4 Posterior triangle of neck with spinal accessory nerve and branches of cervical plexus

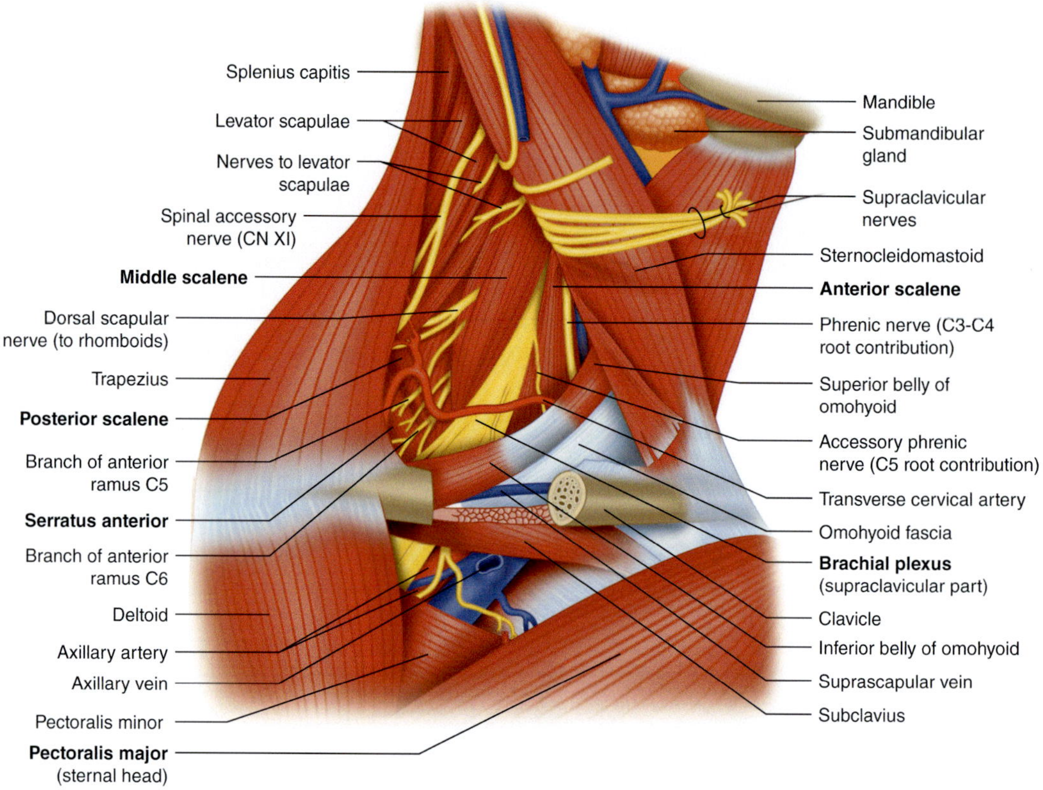

Fig. 4.5 Deeper dissection of posterior triangle illustrating the larger occipital triangle and smaller omoclavicular triangle

Fig. 4.6 Borders of the anterior triangle of the neck

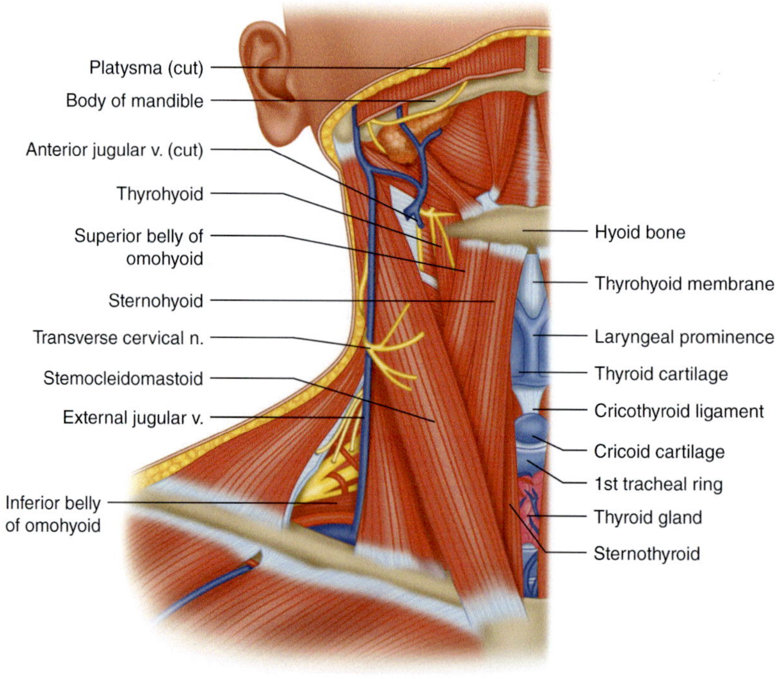

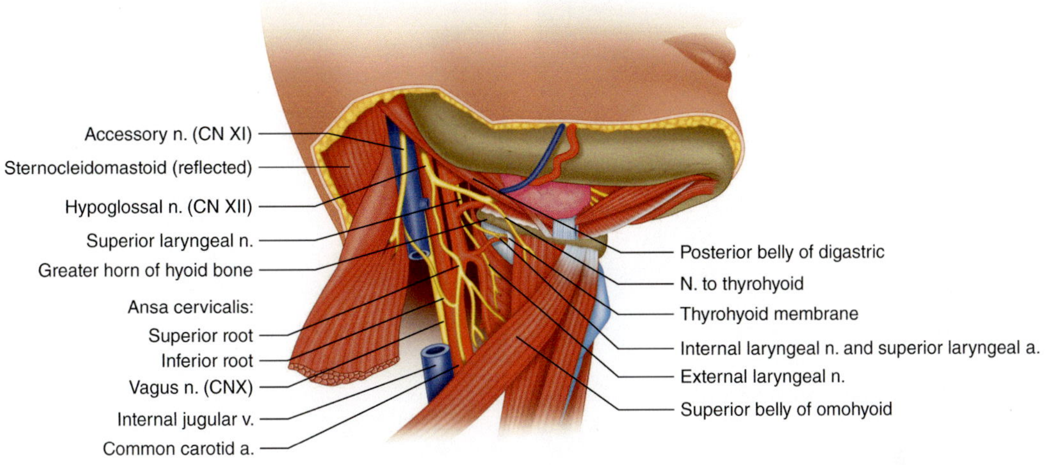

Fig. 4.7 Submental triangle of neck

Skin Incisions

1. Make incisions through the skin only, along the lines indicated in Fig. 4.8.
2. Make an anterior midline incision from the chin to the suprasternal notch (Fig. 4.9).
3. Make an incision along the inferior border of the mandible, from the angle of the mandible to the chin (Fig. 4.10).
4. Make an incision along the anterior border of the clavicle (Fig. 4.11), from the trapezius to the suprasternal notch.
5. For better exposure, you may elect to carry this incision superiorly along the anterior border of the trapezius muscle from the clavicle to the angle of the mandible.

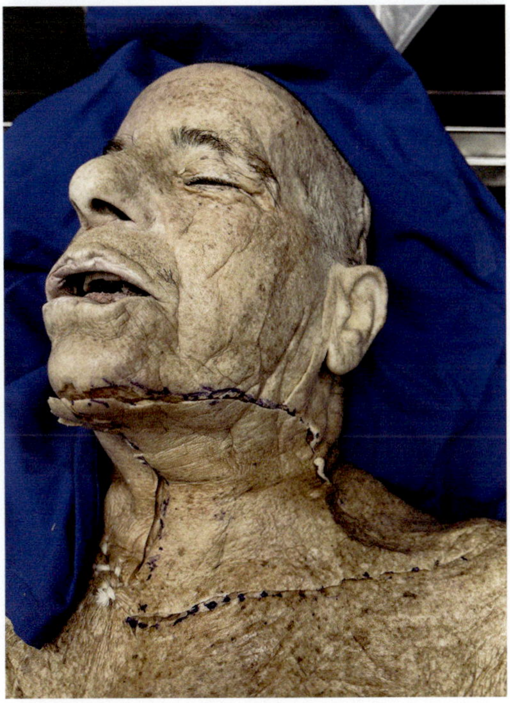

Fig. 4.8 Dotted lines represent incisions for neck exposure

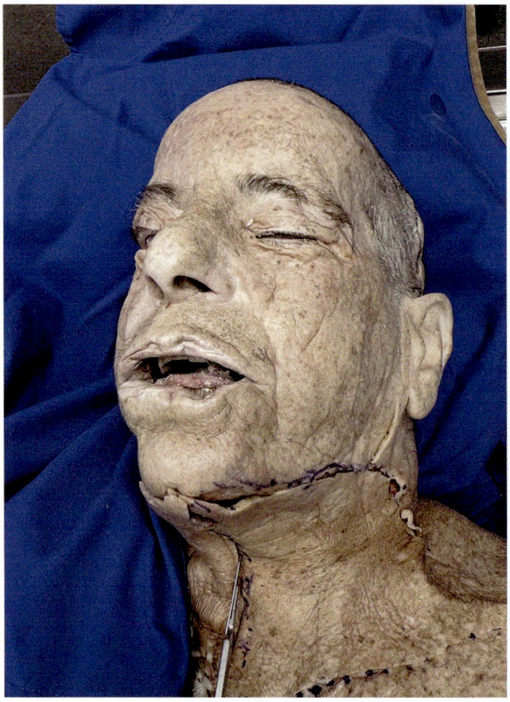

Fig. 4.9 Midline incision from chin (mandible) to suprasternal notch

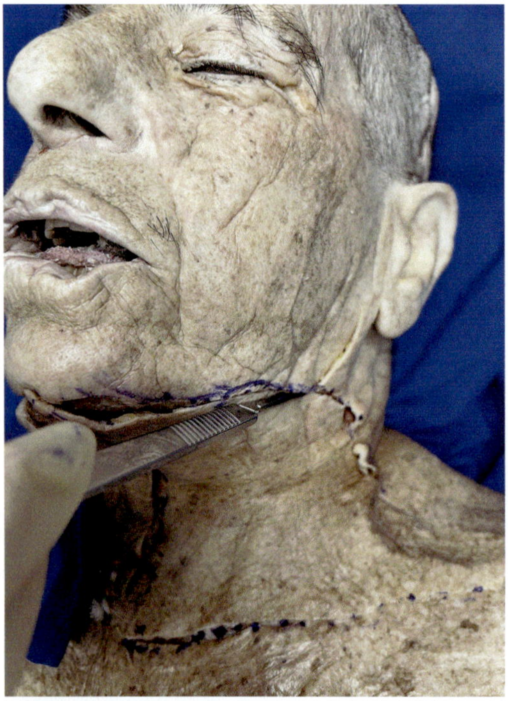

Fig. 4.10 Incision along margin of mandible

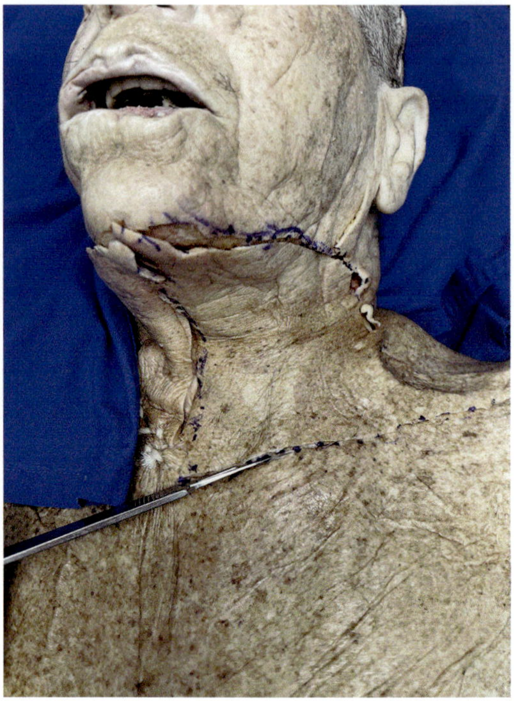

Fig. 4.11 Incision along clavicle

Skin Reflection

1. Beginning at the anterior midline (Fig. 4.12), carefully dissect in the subcutaneous plane in the lateral direction.
2. Identify the sensory supraclavicular nerves passing into the skin (Fig. 4.4). They may be difficult to find as they are easily sacrificed with the skin reflection.
3. Note the underlying subcutaneous fat (Fig. 4.13) and how it varies in thickness.

Clinical Correlation

Submental pre-platysmal fat is the target of liposuction, minimally invasive and invasive cosmetic surgery to reduce fullness under the chin chin, (see Chap. 3 'Surgical Steps Neck' Figs. 3.131 and 3.132).

4. Carefully elevate the subcutaneous fat exposing the platysma muscle (Fig. 4.14). It represents the SMAS in the neck.

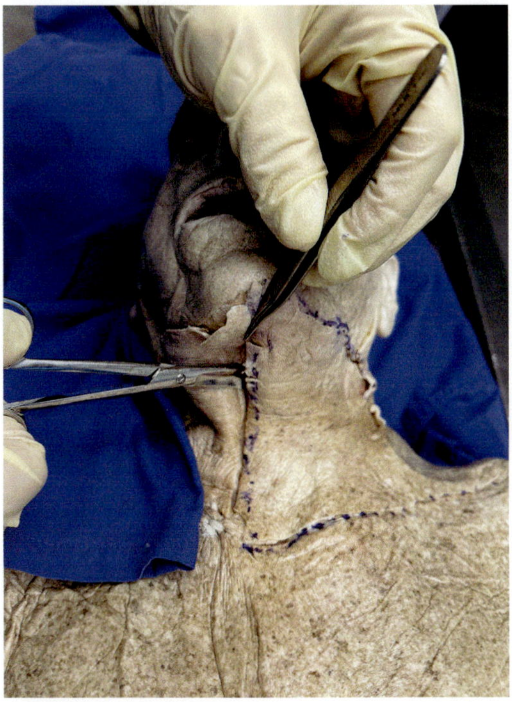

Fig. 4.12 Dissection in subcutaneous plane starting at midline incision

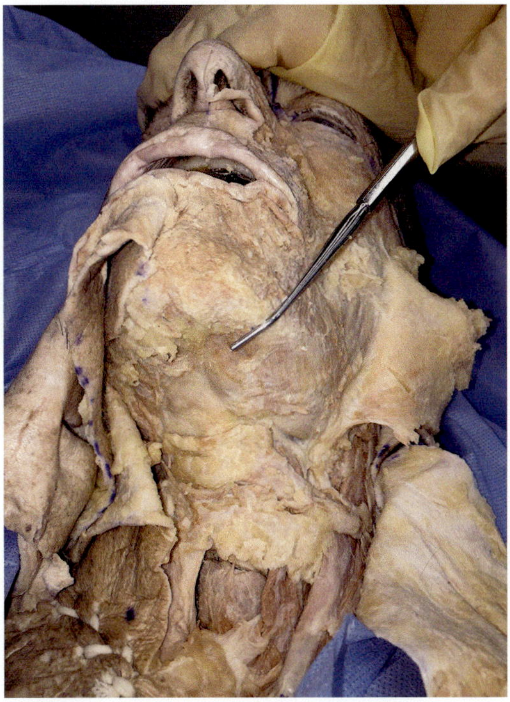

Fig. 4.14 Platysma muscle exposed after reflection of skin flap

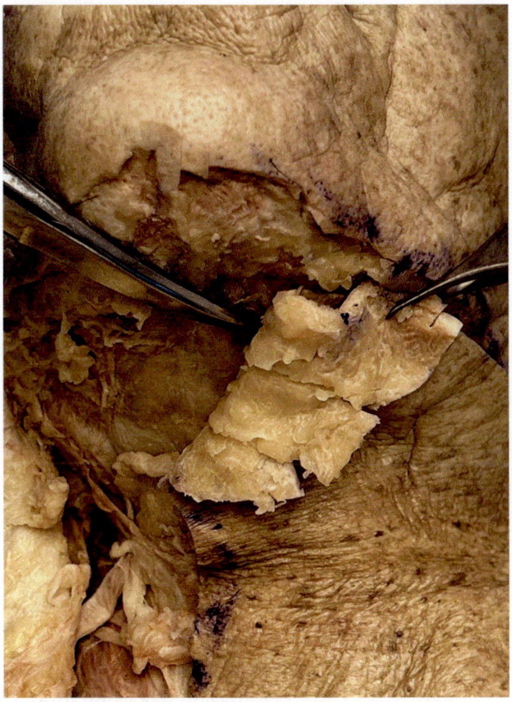

Fig. 4.13 Variable amount of subcutaneous fat is present

The Platysma Muscle

1. Examine the platysma muscle within the superficial fascia. It is a broad sheet of muscle arising from the fascia covering the upper parts of the pectoralis major and deltoid. Further subcutaneous dissection may be necessary for better exposure. Its fibers cross the clavicle and proceed upwards and medially in the neck toward the mandible (Fig. 4.14).
   (a) Ultimately its anterior fibers interlace below the mental symphysis of the chin to join those from the other side of the neck.

Clinical Correlation

With age, the platysma separates into vertically oriented "platysmal bands." To create a more youthful appearance, these separated bands of platysmal muscle are sutured together with anterior platysmal banding surgery. They are also the target for chemodenervation.

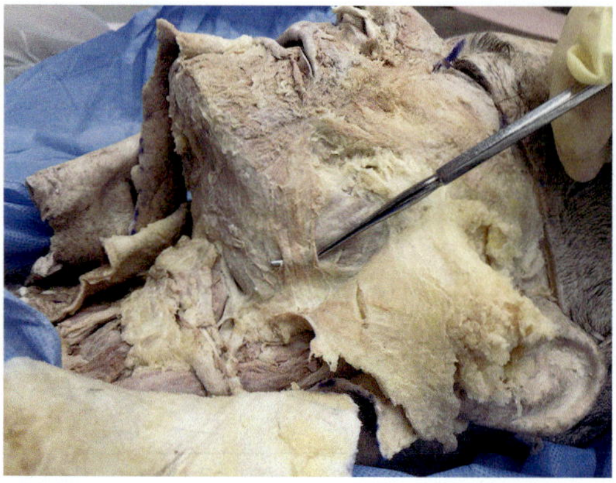

Fig. 4.15 Posterior fibers of platysma crossing mandible and part of masseter muscle

(b) Follow the lateral fibers inserting onto the lower border of the body of the mandible (Fig. 4.14).

(c) Follow the posterior fibers as they cross the mandible and the lower anterior part of the masseter muscle (Fig. 4.15). Their subcutaneous attachments were sacrificed in the dissection of the face.

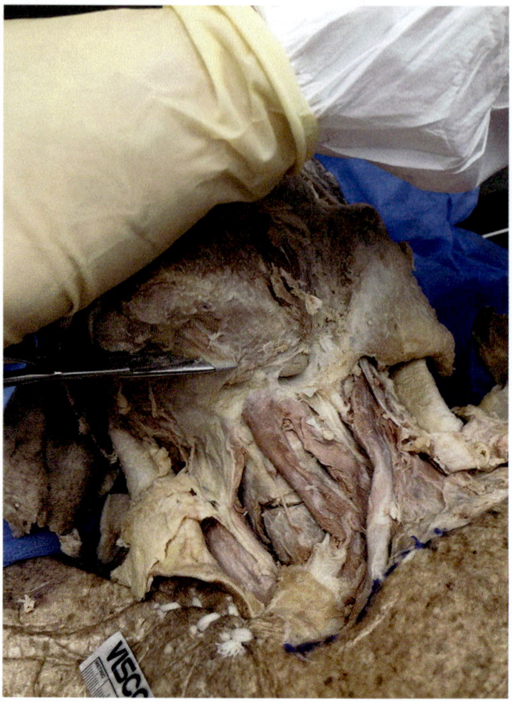

Fig. 4.16 Sharp dissection to free deep aspect of platysma

Clinical Correlations

Contraction of the platysma (a muscle of facial expression) wrinkles the skin of the neck in an oblique fashion. Its anterior portion, which is the thickest, assists in depression of the mandible, lower lip, and angle of the mouth (as with the expression of horror or surprise).

The platysma is innervated by the cervical branch of the facial nerve (CN VII), thus explaining weakness of this muscle in patients with peripheral seventh nerve palsy.

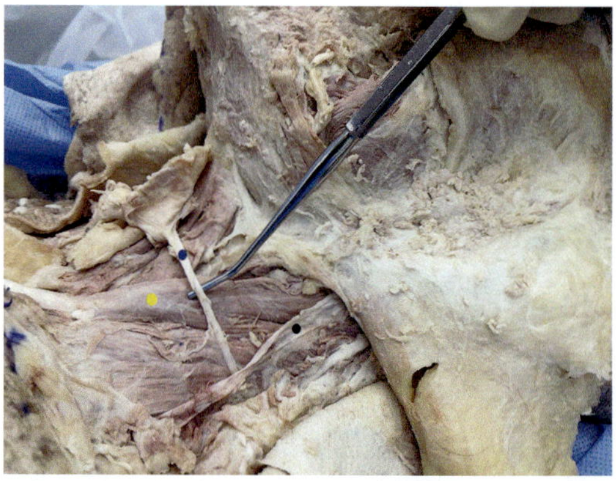

Fig. 4.17 Transverse cervical nerve branch from cervical plexus (blue dot). Note the sternal head (yellow dot)of the sternocleidomastoid muscle, and the jugular vein within the reflected deep cervical fascia (black dot)

Sub-platysma Muscle Dissection

1. Beginning inferior to the mandible carefully use sharp dissection to free the undersurface of the platysma (Fig. 4.16) and attempt to identify the *supra clavicular nerves, and transverse cervical nerve* (Fig. 4.17).
2. Deep (or posterior) to the platysma, note how the SMAS (or superficial cervical fascia) blends with the posterior cervical fascia.
3. Continue careful sub-platysma dissection to identify *the external jugular vein* (Fig. 4.17). The external jugular vein is in the SMAS deep to the platysma. The external jugular vein begins posterior to the angle of the mandible and crosses the superficial surface of the *sternocleidomastoid muscle.* About 3 cm

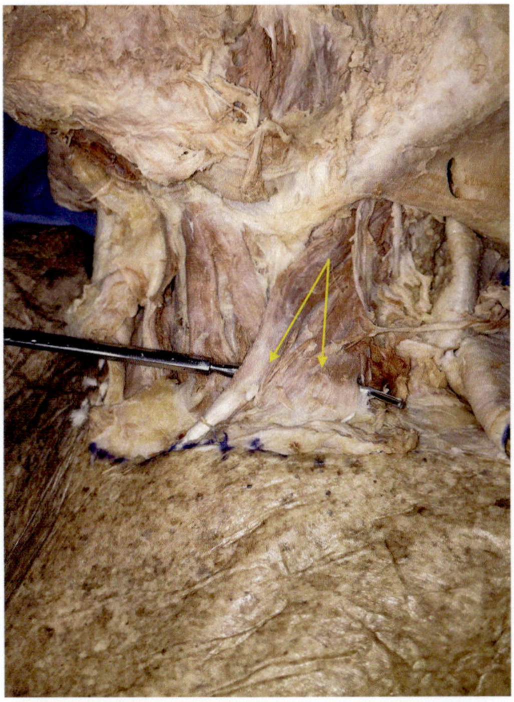

Fig. 4.18 Two heads, depicted by the yellow arrows, of the sternocleidomastoid (SCM) muscle forming posterior border of the anterior cervical triangle

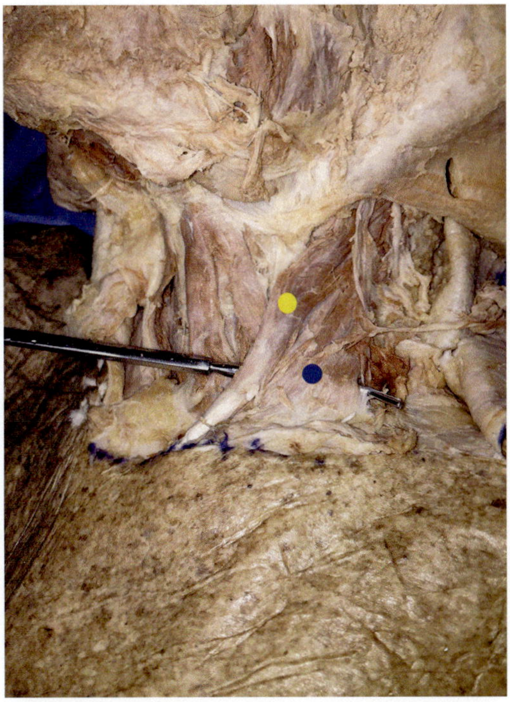

Fig. 4.19 Probe passing deep to sternal (yellow dot) and clavicular (blue dot) heads of SCM

superior to the clavicle, it pierces the investing layer of the deep cervical fascia (roof of the posterior triangle) to drain into *the subclavian vein.*

4. Identify the sternocleidomastoid muscle as it passes obliquely across the side of the neck (Fig. 4.18). This muscle forms the posterior border of the anterior triangle as well as the anterior border of the posterior triangle.
5. Inferiorly, identify the two heads of the sternocleidomastoid muscle (Fig. 4.19):
   (a) The *medial or sternal head* (yellow circle). It is tendinous and attached to the upper part of the anterior surface of the manubrium of the sternum. Trace it as it passes upwards, laterally and posteriorly toward the mastoid process of the temporal bone.
   (b) The *lateral or clavicular head* (blue circle). It is muscular and fibrous. It arises from the upper surface of the medial third of the clavicle. Trace it vertically as it blends with the sternal head.
6. Above, note its tendinous insertion onto the lateral surface of the mastoid process of the temporal bone.
7. Note once again how the sternocleidomastoid muscle divides the side of the neck into the anterior and posterior triangles (Fig. 4.3).
8. Clean its anterior border from the inferior end to its superior attachment on the mastoid process.
9. Near its superior insertion, the sternocleidomastoid muscle may be overlapped by a small portion of the parotid gland. If so, use sharp dissection to free the parotid gland.
10. Using scissors, cut the sternal and clavicular heads of the sternocleidomastoid muscle and reflect the muscle laterally and superiorly (Fig. 4.20). Bluntly dissect it from the fascia that lies deep to it, as far superiorly as the mastoid process.
11. Attempt to conserve the cutaneous branches of the cervical plexus that radiate from the posterior border of the sternocleidomastoid, leaving them attached to the cervical spinal cord (Fig. 4.4).

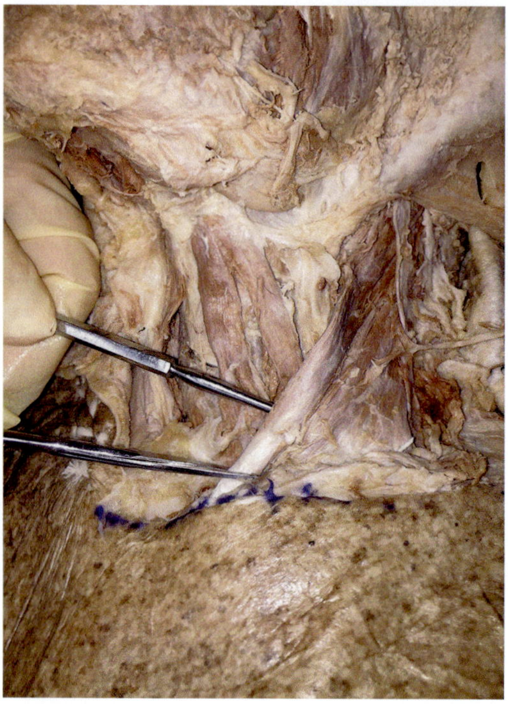

Fig. 4.20 Cutting the sternal and clavicular heads of the SCM

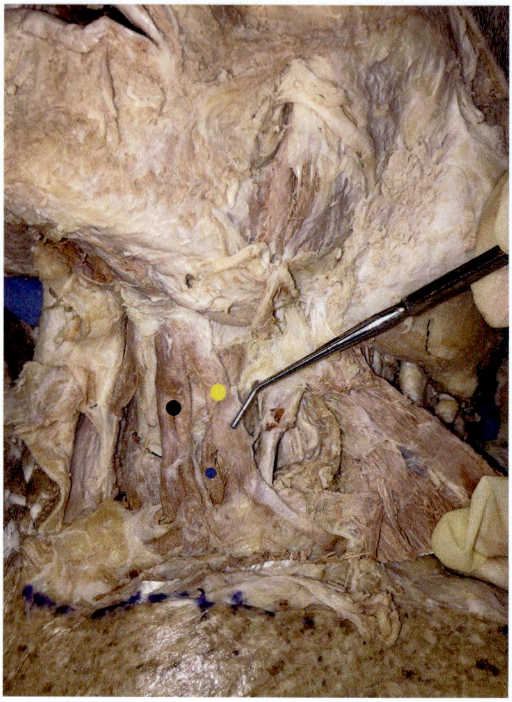

Fig. 4.21 Reflection of SCM reveals superior belly of omohyoid (yellow dot), sternohyoid (black dot), and sternothyroid muscles (blue dot)

12. With the sternocleidomastoid muscle retracted superiorly and laterally, identify the omohyoid, sternohyoid and sternothyroid muscles (Fig. 4.21).
13. Attempt to find the *accessory nerve* (*XI*) where it crosses the deep surface of the sternocleidomastoid near the base of the skull (Fig. 4.4).

Digastric/Submandibular Triangle

1. Carefully remove the fascia from the digastric/submandibular triangle (Fig. 4.3).
2. Identify the submandibular gland, which almost completely fills the triangle and the anterior belly of the digastric muscle (Fig. 4.22).

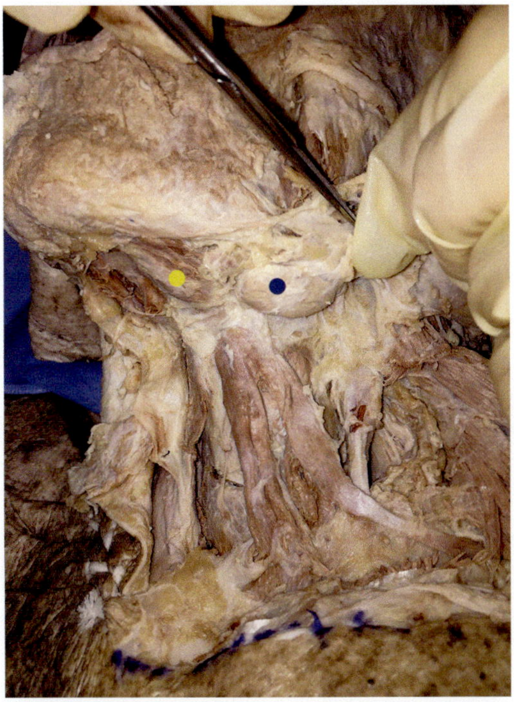

Fig. 4.22 Expose of submandibular gland (blue dot) and anterior belly of digastric (yellow dot) in digastric/submandibular triangle. Note the investing layer of cervical fascia in forceps

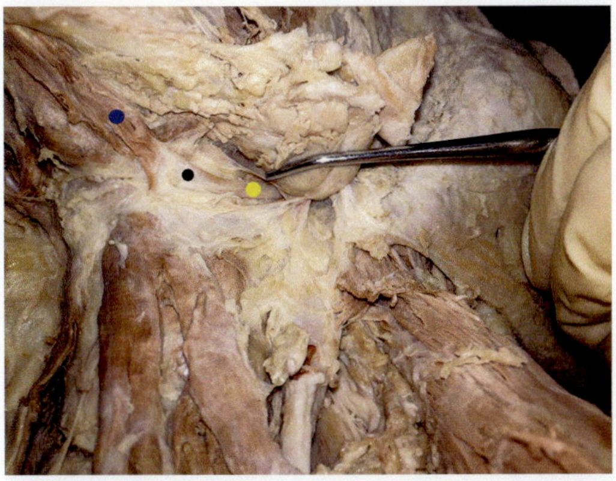

Fig. 4.23 Anterior belly of digastric (blue dot), posterior belly of digastric (yellow dot) and their intermediate tendon (black dot)

3. Displace the submandibular gland superiorly in order to identify the anterior and posterior bellies of the digastric muscles and their intermediate tendon (Fig. 4.23).

Submental Triangle

1. The submental triangle (Fig. 4.3) is an unpaired triangle that crosses the midline. Its boundaries are:

   Right and left: anterior bellies of the right and left digastric muscles.
   Inferior: hyoid bone.
   Superficial (roof): investing layer of the deep cervical fascia (SMAS).
   Deep (floor): mylohyoid muscle.

2. It contains a number of small veins which typically unite to form an anterior jugular vein. The submental triangle also contains a number of submental lymph nodes as well as a variable amount of fat.
3. Following the removal of the deep cervical fascia (SMAS) identify the anterior bellies of the right and left digastric muscles (Figs. 4.24 and 4.25).
4. Use a probe to clean the superficial fascia from the surface of the right and left mylohy-

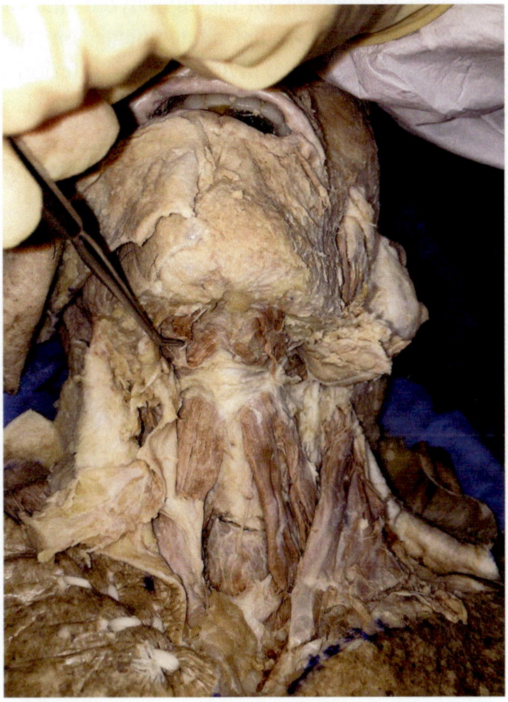

Fig. 4.24 Anterior belly of right digastric muscle

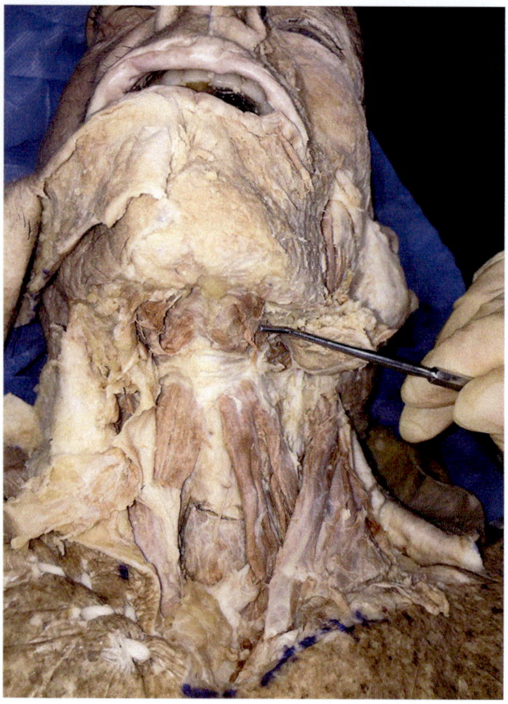

Fig. 4.25 Anterior belly of left digastric muscle

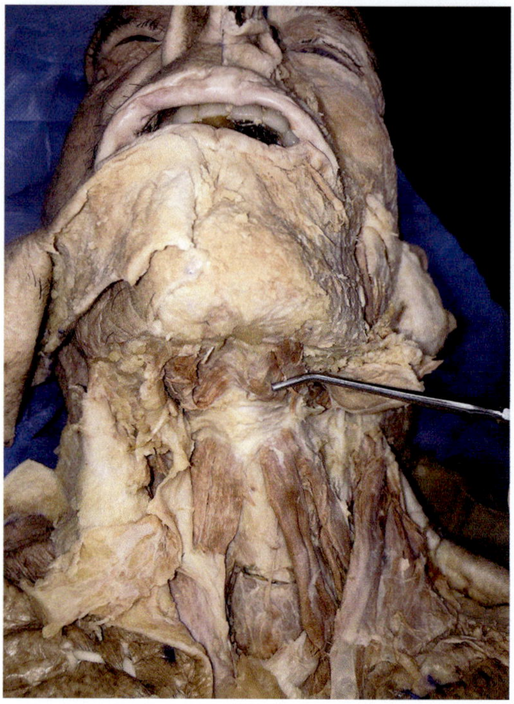

Fig. 4.26. Probe indicates the left mylohyoid muscle

oid muscles. Each mylohyoid muscle has a lateral attachment on the mylohyoid line of the mandible, medial attachments on the midline raphe of the mylohyoid and inferiorly on the hyoid bone (Figs. 4.26 and 4.27). Also identify the hyoid bone (Fig. 4.28).

5. The mylohyoid muscle assist in supporting the floor of the oral cavity.

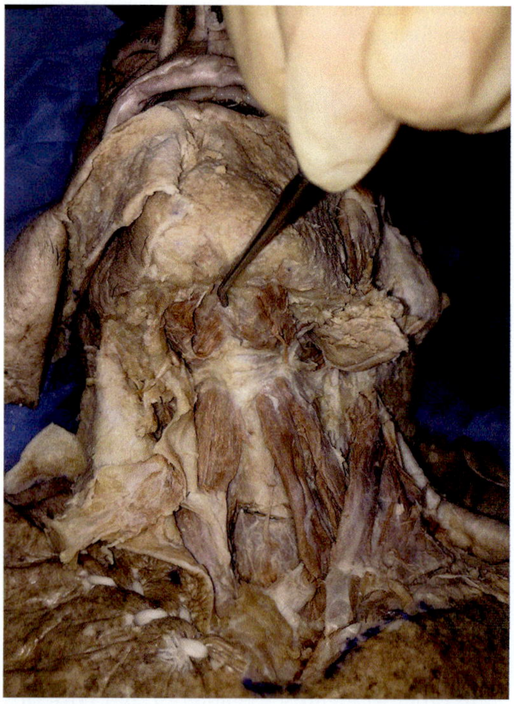

Fig. 4.27 Probe indicates muscular raphe between left and right fibers of the mylohyoid muscles

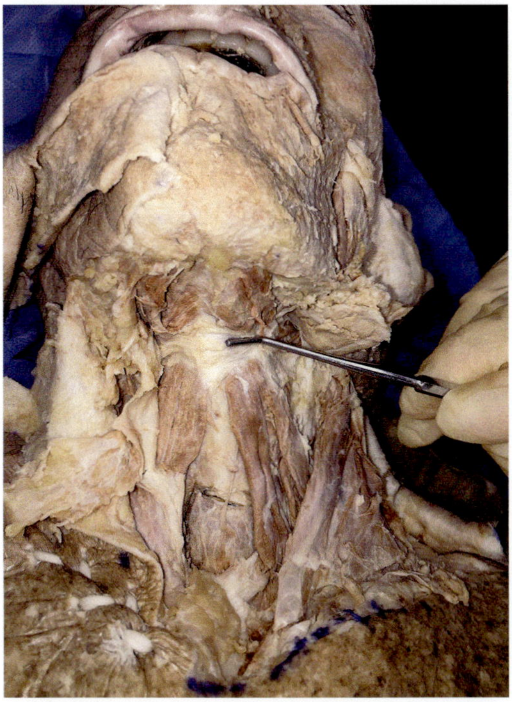

Fig. 4.28 Probe indicates the hyoid bone

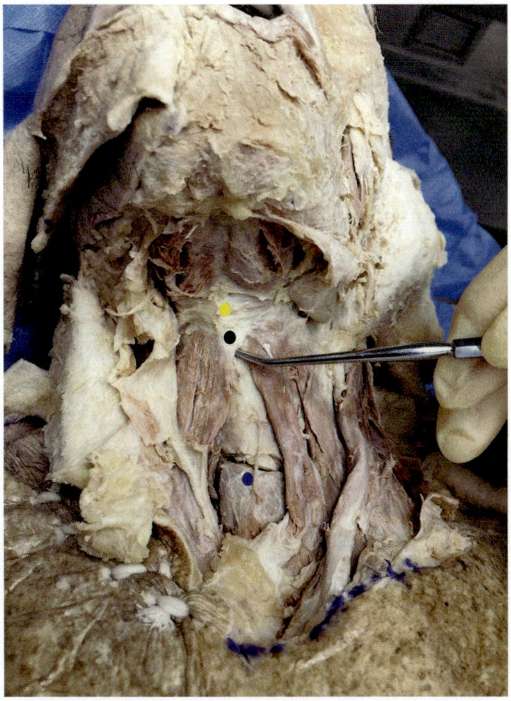

Fig. 4.29 From superior to inferior: hyoid bone (yellow dot), thyrohyoid membrane (black dot), isthmus of thyroid gland (blue dot)

Midline Structures of the Anterior Neck

1. Review the cross-sectional anatomy of the neck (Fig. 4.2).
2. Inferior to the hyoid bone in the midline you should be able to identify the thyrohyoid membrane, trachea and isthmus of the thyroid gland (Fig. 4.29).
3. Note that these structures are bordered laterally on each side by the infrahyoid muscles, i.e., sternohyoid, sternothyroid, and omohyoid.
4. The left lateral lobe of the thyroid gland can be observed by pulling the sternohyoid and sternothyroid in a medial direction (Fig. 4.30).

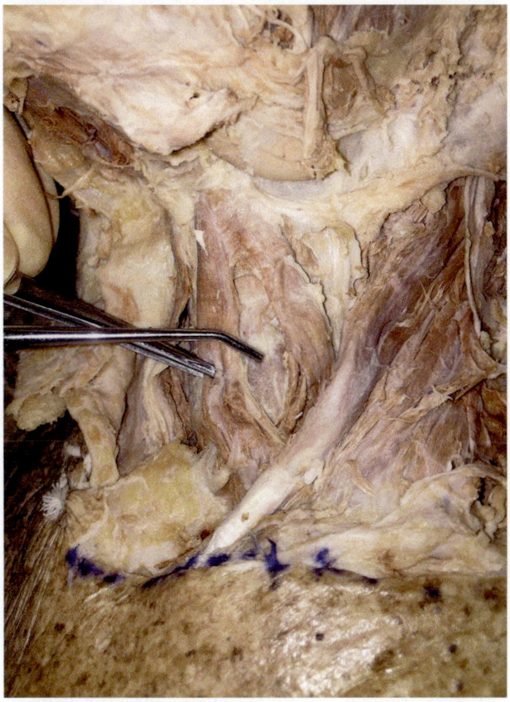

Fig. 4.30 Medial Retraction of sternohyoid and sternothyroid muscles exposes the left lateral lobe of thyroid gland (pointer)

Carotid Triangle of the Anterior Neck

1. The carotid triangle is another subdivision of the anterior triangle of the neck (Fig. 4.3).
2. The borders of this triangle are the anterior border of the SCM, posterior border of the superior belly of the omohyoid and the posterior belly of the digastric muscle. These are depicted with the dotted lines in Fig. 4.31.
3. A number of important structures lie within the carotid triangle, but one of the more important structures is the carotid sheath containing the internal carotid artery, internal jugular vein, and the vagus nerve.
4. Note the fascia of the carotid sheath within the carotid triangle (Fig. 4.32).
5. Earlier you reflected the SCM in a superior and lateral direction which provides you with good access to the carotid triangle and the carotid sheath (Fig. 4.33).

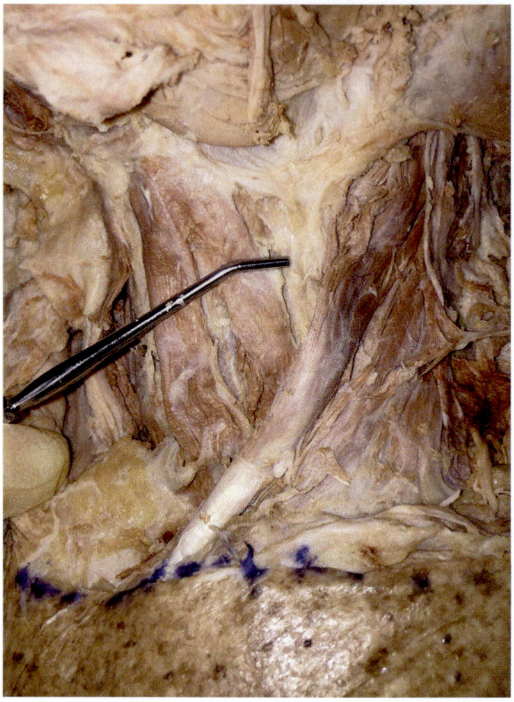

Fig. 4.32 Fascia within the carotid triangle covering carotid sheath

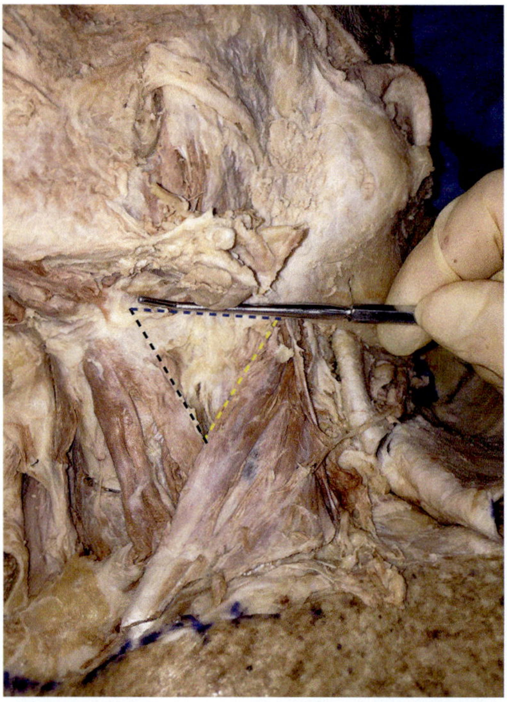

Fig. 4.31 Borders of carotid triangle: posterior belly of digastric (blue dashes), anterior border of SCM (yellow dashes), and posterior border of superior belly of omohyoid (black dashes)

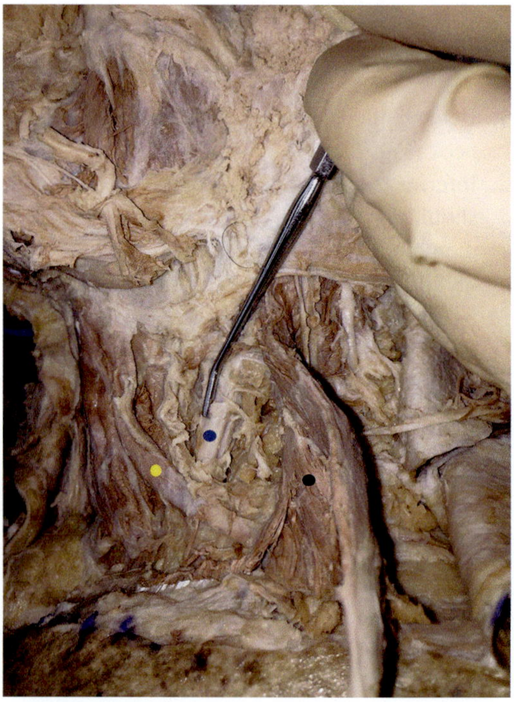

Fig. 4.33 Reflecting the SCM (black dot) in a superolateral direction yields good access to the carotid sheath (blue dot); yellow dot is superior belly of omohyoid

6. Once you have opened the carotid sheath, retract the internal jugular vein in a medial direct. This maneuver will provide you good access to the common carotid artery and the vagus nerve as shown in Fig. 4.34.

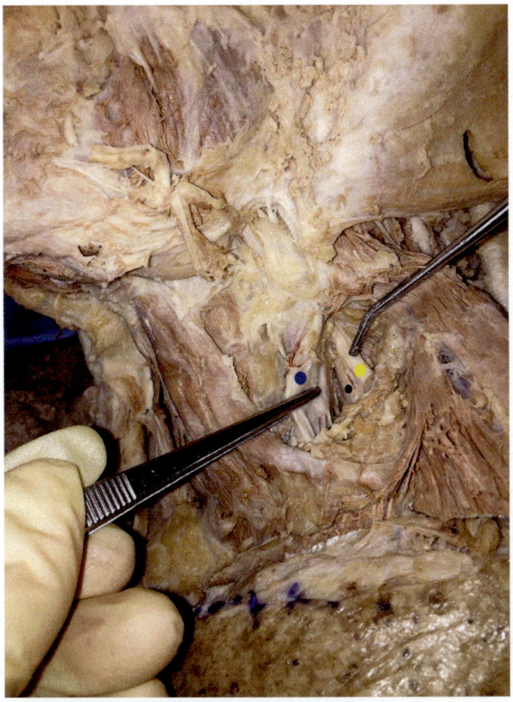

Fig. 4.34 Retraction of internal jugular vein (blue dot) medially yields good exposure of the common carotid artery (yellow dot) and the vagus nerve (black dot)

Surgical Neck Lift

Surgical approach to the neck involves a thorough understanding of the anatomy, terminology and danger zones as described, and dissected in this chapter. Another cadaver is needed for an exercise of anatomic dissection for a subcutaneous neck lift with platysma plication. Since a neck lift is often performed in conjunction with a face lift, it is included toward the end of Chap. 3 of this manual in section "Deep plane/ Biplanar Face lift", Surgical steps : Neck.

The exercise is meant to complement, not replace a comprehensive surgical facelift and neck lift course or an oculofacial plastic, facial plastic, comprehensive plastic or surgical cosmetic fellowship.

Further Reading

Gosling JA, Harris PF, Whitmore I, Willan PLT. Human anatomy color atlas and text. 4th ed. St. Louis: Mosby Publishing; 2002. p. 284–327.

Hiatt JL, Gartner LP. Textbook of head & neck anatomy. 4th ed. Philadelphia: Lippincott Williams & Wilkins; 2010. p. 104–36.

Janviz J, Nadol JB Jr, Galla RJ, Fabian RL, Montgomery WW. Surgical anatomy of the head and neck. Philadelphia: Lippincott Williams & Wilkins.; 2001. p. 507–674.

McMinn RMH, Hutchings RT, Logan BM. Colar atlas of head and neck anatomy. Chicago: Year Book Medical Publishers, Inc.; 1981.

Rosse C, Gaddum-Rosse P. Hollinsheads's textbook of anatomy. 5th ed. Philadelphia: Lippincott-Raven; 1997. p. 707–30.

Index

E. H. Bedrossian Jr et al. (eds.), *Anatomy of the Forehead, Face, and Neck*,
https://doi.org/10.1007/978-3-031-56140-5

MIX
Papier aus verantwortungsvollen Quellen
Paper from responsible sources
FSC® C105338

If you have any concerns about our products,
you can contact us on
ProductSafety@springernature.com

In case Publisher is established outside the EU,
the EU authorized representative is:
Springer Nature Customer Service Center GmbH
Europaplatz 3, 69115 Heidelberg, Germany

Printed by Libri Plureos GmbH
in Hamburg, Germany